CW01475594

Anne Simons

Living Longer in Good Health Through OPCs

The standard work on the subject of OPCs

Can red wine reduce the risk of heart attack? What does scurvy have to do with OPCs? How do we know that OPCs is 100 percent bioavailable? Why do OPCs increase the effect of vitamin C tenfold? Are OPCs the long sought-after 'vitamin P'? How does oxygen develop into dangerous free radicals that cause various diseases? And how do OPCs prevent our cells from becoming 'rancid'? Anne Simons explains clinical studies in an exciting and generally understandable way and allows her readers to share the information and thoughts that Professor Masquelier entrusted to her during detailed discussions. The users of OPCs, who have experienced relief or healing of various diseases and impairments through the natural remedy, also have their say in case studies. Why are OPCs also considered an anti-aging vitamin? How do OPCs prevent atherosclerosis and arteriosclerosis? How can OPCs strengthen and heal in various areas, such as concentration and visual impairment, wounds and bone fractures, skin problems, hormonal disorders, headaches, inflammation and allergies? How can OPCs reduce wrinkles and maintain smooth, fresh skin in the long term? How can the vital substance be used in animals? You can find out all about OPCs in this standard reference work.

Anne Simons has popularized the vital substance OPCs in German-speaking countries. Hundreds of thousands of people have read her books on the powerful anti-aging vitamin. Her detailed knowledge of OPCs comes from first-hand experience: until his death in 2009, Anne Simons was a close friend of Professor Dr. Jack Masquelier, who discovered OPCs and researched it for decades. The author studied humanities and has published non-fiction books on numerous health issues and related topics.

Anne Simons

Living Longer in Good Health Through OPCs

The Natural Active Substances for the New Millennium

MayaMedia

Disclaimer
Every effort has been made to insure that the information provided in this book is accurate and can be useful in promoting good health. It is, however, not meant to replace medical advice or support. This book is intended to provide readers with guidance for the care and self-treatment of everyday disorders. The authors and the publisher assume no liability for potential damage resulting from the use or abuse of the material presented in this book.

This book is partly based on the German book "Gesund länger leben durch OPC", MayaMedia Verlag Dr. Andreas Gößling, © 1999-2025

Data according to GPSR:
MayaMedia Verlag Dr. Andreas Gößling, Ringstr. 93, D-14612 Falkensee, office@mayamedia.de

Illustrations in the book by courtesy of Alfa Omega, Rome
Book setting and cover: Adobe InDesign by MayaMedia
Printing: Libri Plureos GmbH, Friedensallee 273, 22763 Hamburg
ISBN: 978-3-944488-65-3

Table of Contents

Foreword

Nowadays a trend can be observed which at first glance may seem paradoxical: although human life expectancy has dramatically increased during the last one hundred years and medicine has recorded unprecedented technical progress, the subject of health is gaining increasing importance for many people. Instead of blindly relying on these grand achievements, people are taking control of their own health care, obtaining information about alternative healing methods and displaying a great interest in a 'healthy diet' as well as nutritional supplements. The market is booming.

Upon closer examination, we find that this development is not all that paradoxical. In statistical terms, our life expectancy has lengthened impressively, but, unfortunately, the period of time during which we enjoy good health has not increased proportionately. Symptoms of wear and exhaustion, especially in connection with a gradually degenerating immune system, manifest themselves in the course of time and severely impair our quality of life. What good is a long life expectancy if you spend half the time suffering pain and exhaustion or if you have to forego all pleasures! Our high-tech medicine is - with some luck - able to 'repair' the worst cases, but physical breakdown, surgery and rehabilitation are linked to dramatic turning points in the affected person's life: in all probability, life after such an event is no longer what it used to be; in most cases it is impossible to continue as 'before'.

In view of this unpleasant notion - which unfortunately is grim reality for many people - we had better take preventive action, look for nutrients, vitamins and wholesome lifestyles in order to minimize health risks.

The search for the fountain of youth is a subject that is as old as the history of mankind: are there any substances that will keep us young and healthy for a long time?

This may sound rather audacious, but I nevertheless dare claim that they may indeed have been discovered, substances offered by nature which can spare us disease and ailing, even premature aging our whole life long ...

'OPCs' is the abbreviation for oligomeric proanthocyanidins. These are natural substances existing in numerous plants ... and in red wine. Their healing effects have been known for centuries, but the actual substances to which these effects are attributable have only been discovered and systematically explored in the twentieth century. Multi-faceted tests conducted according to strict scientific criteria have revealed amazing details: OPCs are the strongest antioxidants presently known, 18 times stronger than vitamin C and 40 to 50 times stronger than vitamin E! They have tremendous vasculo-protective properties, and are thus an important factor in the struggle against cardiovascular diseases, arteriosclerosis, heart attack and stroke. They lower the cholesterol level. Their collagen-enhancing properties result in numerous health benefits. They protect the skin - as well as all other body tissue - against rapid aging and wrinkle formation and they help to preserve a youthful appearance much longer.

Inflammation, allergic reactions, tooth decay, failing vision, lack of concentration and age-related cerebral disorders ... the list is extensive. I can only recommend that you form your own opinion: obtain information about OPCs and take them.

And rest assured that reputable scientists, pre-eminently Professor Jack Masquelier, have been investigating this substance, for more than 60 years. In France it has been used as the basis for three vasoprotective drugs prescribed by physicians since 1950.

Masquelier was the pioneer in this field. His research has been systematically documented by

Bert Schwitters, the renowned author of numerous books and articles on health and nutrition topics. In his books *OPC in Practice* and *A Lifetime Devoted to OPC*, all research results have been collected and presented in a manner which even a layperson can easily understand: a comprehensive presentation of all the scientific literature on OPCs. I am grateful to Bert Schwitters. He granted me access to essential information. And I am deeply grateful to Professor Masquelier himself, an outstanding scientist and wonderful teacher, who answered my questions with the utmost patience.

Now let us embark on a thrilling voyage to the substances that may revolutionize our health: OPCs for living longer in good health.

Introduction (2017):
My 20 years with OPCs

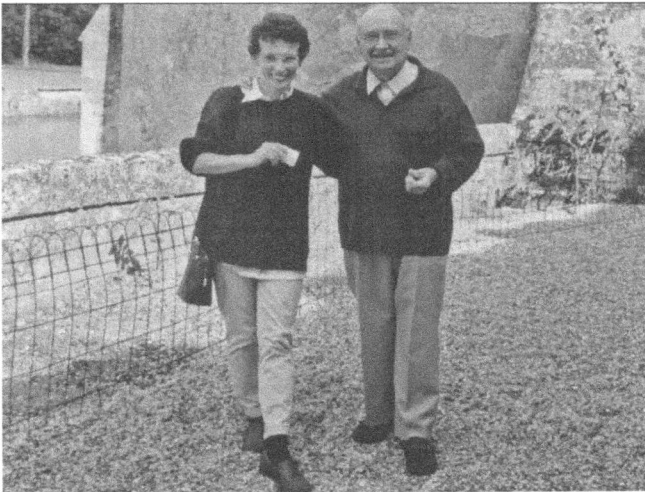

More than 20 years have now passed since I came across OPCs and wrote my first book on the subject (published in 1998 under the title *Das OPC-Gesundheitsbuch* by Scherz-Verlag) - time for a look back.

The beginning

When I first saw the list of applications for the natural remedy OPCs in the mid-1990s and was asked by a publisher to research the subject for a book project, I spontaneously declined. A panacea that is supposed to help from head to toe, from harmless complaints to serious civilisation diseases? That couldn't be serious. So I thought.

A little later, I came across OPCs again, this time while researching the 'French paradox'. This is a statistical phenomenon: in the middle of the 20th century, it was discovered that the French had the lowest risk of cardiac death in the world, even though they lived unhealthier lives than other peoples, i.e. they smoked, did little sport, ate a lot of fat and regularly drank red wine.

Now my interest was piqued. I researched and found highly interesting studies and research results on OPCs, an essential ingredient in red wine, and got to know their discoverer, the French scientist Professor Dr Jack Masquelier.

My own first experience

In the meantime, I had been taking 50 mg of OPCs daily for a year - after all, the extensive study of the new substance also required a self-test. A random dental examination with x-rays after this year showed that my gums, which had receded due to severe periodontal disease, and my jawbone, which had deteriorated, had rebuilt. Just like that.

This exciting experience was the beginning of a journey through a scientific field in which botany, in particular the healing properties of plants, and human physiology combine in a fascinating way.

The explorer

My friendship with Professor Masquelier

I had the great good fortune to meet Professor Masquelier, the discoverer and researcher of OPCs, in person and to be able to work with him. Over the years, a wonderful friendship developed between him, his wife and myself, which lasted until his death in 2009.

Professor Masquelier was a very fine man, highly educated, respectful and dignified, a sensitive character, a teacher much appreciated by his students and a brilliant scientist. He was a doctor of natural sciences, a title that no longer exists due to its almost unmanageable complexity, as it encompassed biology, chemistry, biochemistry, pharmacy and medicine.

Why was I able to meet Professor Masquelier? As a successful author of naturopathic non-fiction books in Germany, I had thoroughly familiarised myself with the subject of OPCs, and I also speak English and French in addition to my native German. This meant that I met the requirements for writing a book focussing on Jack Masquelier's research into OPCs.

The decisive factor, however, was that the professor and I got on well from the very beginning and maintained a personal, friendly dialogue that went beyond our work together. Shortly before his death, I received a touching letter from him and, 'as proof of my friendship', a 546-page autobiography, *Un Enseignant d'Autrefois* (A teacher as they used to be), which he had had printed in small numbers for his family and close friends. In addition to describing his academic work, it contains private anecdotes and is a source of personal details from his life as well as a stylistically outstanding document of contemporary French history. I keep this one copy like a treasure!

What many scientists before Jack Masquelier, including two-time Nobel Prize winner Alfred Szent-György, failed to achieve, became his life's success: the discovery of the colourless substance OPCs and the research into them, which Professor Masquelier pursued with passion throughout his life.

Jack Masquelier - a biographical survey

In a small town in the north of France, there was a 'Masquelier' street named not after the famous researcher, but after his father. After the First World War, Arthur Masquelier rebuilt the destroyed houses in the northern French towns where the young family then lived.

Early fascination with nature

Born in Paris on 14 April 1922, Jack, whose English spelling of his name was due to his mother's Anglophilia, already had a wide range of interests as a child. He could read and write at the age of four, immersed himself in literature and equally in nature: animals, plants, minerals. He learnt Latin and Greek. He examined the fascinating structure of plants under a microscope and organised shells and other sea creatures collected on the beach into a systematic order. He was an exceptional pupil right from the start, and his teacher Abbé Moronval gave him the task of organising the maritime collection of the museum in Malo when he was still in fifth grade.

As a secondary school pupil, he deepened his knowledge of chemistry in his own laboratory. He was also responsible for managing the school science collection. In 1938, at the request of his school, he wrote what was probably the first of his more than 200 scientific publications, in which he described how to create a shell collection according to scientific standards.

Forced labour in Erfurt

After graduating from high school with honours in 1939, Jack Masquelier, who also achieved top marks throughout his studies in medicine and pharmacy, had a great career ahead of him. But history initially had other plans: War, deportation to Erfurt and forced labour in a pharmacy there. Due to the war, there was a shortage of medical personnel in Hitler's Germany, which is why young specialists from abroad were forcibly recruited to work in hospitals and pharmacies.

Only towards the end of the war, after an adventurous escape back to Bordeaux, was Jack Masquelier able to complete his pharmacy studies there with a doctoral thesis on the oligomeric procyanidins (OPCs) he had discovered. He again achieved the top grade of 'Très honorable' ('Highly honourable') in the rare and very demanding field of natural sciences, 'es-sciences'. This was to be the beginning of a lifetime of research into OPCs.

Rapid career of a natural scientist

At the age of just 27, Dr Masquelier became the youngest member of the Faculty of Pharmacy and taught microbiology and plant biochemistry. At the same time, he conducted research into wine and health and published a ground-breaking essay on the antibacterial effect of wine, which also helped Masquelier to achieve fame outside France (*'Le vin dans l'alimentation humaine'*). This was followed by a chair in oenology (wine science). In 1956, he was appointed professor in the medically orientated 'Matière Médicale' department in Bordeaux. In 1957, he became Vice Dean of the Faculty of Medicine and Pharmacy, in 1963, Professor of Phytochemistry at the University of Laval in Quebec, and from 1970 until his retirement in 1984, he was Dean of the Faculty of Pharmacy at the University of Bordeaux.

Developing natural medicines

Professor Masquelier was the official expert for drug analyses for the French Ministry of Health. He himself developed a number of medicinal products authorised in France, not only on the basis of OPCs. He was also far ahead of his time in researching intestinal bacteria, which is highly topical today: he developed the drug *Lactiflore,* which helped to make the intake of antibiotics tolerable for the intestinal flora back in the early 1960s.

However, his name will remain associated above all with OPCs. Jack Masquelier is the father of this phenomenal protective substance that brings health, healing and quality of life to people all over the world well into old age.

Why are OPCs not better known?

Like many great discoveries, OPCs only found their way into the global public consciousness gradually and in a roundabout way. In contrast to vitamin C, which was discovered two decades earlier, it has not yet been recognised as the most powerful plant antioxidant and vitamin P in the scientific canon. Why is that?

There are a whole range of reasons why oligomeric procyanidins are not mentioned on an equal footing with vitamin C as a collagen-protecting and antioxidant substance, although their antiradical effect is much stronger.

Linguistic inconsistency

Linguistic inconsistency is one of the reasons. For two centuries, scientists have been searching for the colourless oligomeric procyanidins. Among them were the chemist couple Lord and Lady Robinson, the German chemist Otto Rosenheim and the Nobel Prize winner Albert Szent-Györgyi. They all labelled the substance they were looking for with their own - and always different - term. Throughout the history of research, oligomeric procyanidins (OPCs) have been called 'chromogen', 'leucocyanin', 'proanthocyanidins' or 'pycnogenol'. These are polyphenols with a flavanic core, which chemically belong to the flavanols, but are usually referred to imprecisely as 'bioflavonoids' or 'grape seed extract'.

The whole world knows OPCs, but nobody knows that this is what they are!

In contrast to the flavanols, i.e. OPCs, the 'bioflavonoids' are not 'bio' at all, as they are hardly or not at all bioavailable. The term 'grape seed extract' says nothing about the OPCs content. In fact, when 'newly discovered' healthy medicinal plants and fruits (such as cranberries) are promoted these days, they are actually 'flavanols', i.e. OPCs. Their favourable health effects are attributed to their high content of 'bioflavonoids', whereas in reality they are 'flavanols', i.e. OPCs. The whole world knows OPCs, but nobody knows that this is what they are!

In the wrong place at the wrong time

Another reason for OPCs' still low profile is that Masquelier was way ahead of his time. OPCs were discovered in the wrong place at the wrong time: after the war - when Europe was preoccupied with other topics - and in France, not in the USA. Most of Professor Masquelier's publications on OPCs appeared in France in French, which makes it difficult for the world to know and research them.

The international scientific language is English. Masquelier's studies were published in the pre-Google era and are almost impossible to find on the Internet. And for many people, what cannot be found on the Internet does not exist.

Pioneering publications

Yet there are plenty of ground-breaking international publications that drew attention to OPCs as early as the 1980s and 1990s. Here is just a small selection: in 1987, Professor Masquelier received a patent in the USA for the anti-radical effect of OPCs and their medical and cosmetic use. It explicitly states that OPCs provide a method for 'preventing and combating the harmful biological effects of free radicals in the organism of warm-blooded animals and especially humans; namely cerebral involution [age-related brain regression processes], hypoxia [lack of oxygen supply to the tissue] after atherosclerosis, heart and brain infarction, tumour development, inflammation, ischaemia [reduced blood flow or complete lack of blood flow to a tissue], changes in joint fluid and collagen degradation.'

In the same year, the Japanese biologist Uchida published a study according to which the anti-radical effect of OPCs is fifty times stronger than that of vitamin E. In 1993, it was proven (Frenkel et al.) that the antioxidants in wine inhibit the oxidation of human LDL cholesterol. Two years later, Serge Renaud and others proved that OPCs prevent platelet aggregation.

How is it possible that these overwhelming results, although now published in English and in international journals, did not have a greater impact and went unnoticed by the US Food and Drug Administration (FDA), which is responsible for food monitoring and drug approval? After all, this agency is responsible for US public health. Is it perhaps because OPCs are purely herbal, whereas the FDA is primarily concerned with monitoring new synthetic products?

Every dietary supplement needs its own scientific studies

Scientific acceptance in this country is made more difficult by the fact that many OPCs products are now offered as dietary supplements. According to European law, however, scientific studies must be carried out for each product that is claimed to have healing effects. However, very few fulfil this requirement. For legal reasons, the evidence for the physiological effects of the French OPCs drug *Endotélon* provided in scientific studies cannot simply be claimed for other OPCs preparations such as food supplements - even if these naturally have healing effects due to their OPCs content.

OPCs in German-speaking countries

My books and numerous lectures have popularised OPCs in German-speaking countries. Initially I spoke to 20 interested people, but by now the topic fills town halls. My lecture is available online as a video (www.mayamedia.de). Over the past two decades, knowledge of OPCs has spread, particularly as a result of people having good experiences and telling others about them.

I have received countless, sometimes dramatic and very touching testimonials on the fringes of lectures in which OPCs played a key role. I have collected and published these reports, for example in the German e-book *Das OPC-Wunderbuch*.

Grateful diabetics

OPCs have proven to be an important protective substance for diabetics. Diabetics have a disturbed sugar metabolism, which has a negative effect on the vascular wall. This is susceptible to increased degradation. One of the long-term consequences of diabetes is the collapse of the entire vascular system, which can lead to serious illnesses. Degeneration of the heart arteries can lead to heart attacks, degeneration of the brain arteries to strokes and degeneration of the leg arteries to gangrene. In extreme cases, toes and the lower sections of the leg have to be amputated.

Diabetics are also prone to atherosclerosis. Diabetes must therefore be regarded as a vascular disease with all the associated complications. This is also impressively demonstrated by the statistical figures. Well over two thirds of all diabetics die from a heart attack or stroke.

In the capillary microcirculation, other organs are

also affected by the vascular damage. The kidneys can degenerate to the point of failure. Capillary problems impair eye function ('diabetic retinopathy'), sometimes to the point of blindness.

The collapse of the vascular system is therefore one of the main late effects of diabetes. OPCs are the ideal natural active ingredient for their vasoprotective properties. By fulfilling the role of vitamin P, they prevent the dangerous permeability of blood vessels. Diabetics regularly tell me that they feel healthier since taking OPCs.

OPCs play no role in maintaining normal blood sugar and are therefore not a substitute for insulin. However, they are very important in diabetes because of their role in maintaining the vascular system. In this context, OPCs have been thoroughly researched in France, particularly in the case of diabetic retinopathy, as described in this book.

New research

Since the era of Masquelier's own research, numerous other scientific studies on OPCs have been published. Many of them confirm the results that the professor and his colleagues had already achieved 50 years earlier, for example with regard to the collagen-protecting effect of OPCs, the reduction of LDL cholesterol and the corresponding reduction in heart attacks.

OPCs optimise bodily functions

There is a study from Maastricht University from 2011 (Antje R. Weseler et al: *Pleiotropic Benefit of Monomeric and Oligomeric Flavanols on Vascular Health - A Randomised Controlled Clinical Pilot Study*) I would like to highlight here because it provides the scientific background for a phenomenon that seems unspectacular at first glance, namely how to stay healthy with OPCs.

Sometimes I have conversations that go something like this: Someone says to me, 'Now I've been taking OPCs for a year (or two or more years) and I don't notice any change at all.' Then I ask back: 'Are you suffering from a disease?' - 'No.' - 'Do you have any complaints?' - 'No.' - 'So you're healthy and doing well?' - 'Yes.'

Of course, maintaining the health that you have and have always had is not as noticeable as a cure where you noticeably change from a bad condition and body feeling to a good one.

Sometimes I also hear from people who, in the course of taking OPCs, gradually experience an improvement in a suboptimal condition without realising it. At some point they realise that a bronchitis (or some other problem) that used to occur every year has now not occurred for three years. The Dutch study provides an interesting explanation for this - homeostasis.

OPCs work in two ways: as a medicine (they have been prescribed as such by doctors in France for decades) and as a food (supplement). What does this mean?

Specific and non-specific mode of action of OPCs

Medicines and foods have different effects on the body. While a medicine acts specifically on one aspect, such as an enzyme or a receptor, thus producing a strong, rapid effect, our foods, provided they contain all the necessary vitamins, trace elements, minerals and essential fatty acids, ensure long-term, lasting health or maintenance of health. The biologically active substances act slowly and cannot be clearly defined - and yet their deficiency would sooner or later lead to illness. The bioactive ingredients in food exert non-specific, diverse and subtle effects and increase the body's ability to adapt to changes. They support its 'homeostasis'.

Homeostasis - what does it mean?

There are many definitions of homeostasis. They essentially boil down to the fact that the body, which is constantly exposed to internal fluctuations as well as external, including adverse influences, must constantly react to them in order to maintain its performance in all organ systems and in all cells. This constant adaptation to changes represents a fine adjustment that serves to optimise the body. It is about maintaining the inner balance of the organism by adapting the physiological processes to changes.

Homeostasis is a prerequisite for the body's ability to survive. If you consider, for example, the small temperature corridor in which the human body can live, it is actually a miracle that humanity has survived at all. The same applies to every single human life, which over the course of several decades has to cope with an immense remodelling of the body on a cellular level as well as illnesses, injuries, etc. We owe our survival above all to our body's ability to react to changing conditions with the smallest and most subtle corrections.

OPCs help the body to maintain optimum health

What do OPCs have to do with homeostasis? The study by Antje Weseler and colleagues shows that OPCs help the body to adapt dynamically to new circumstances, increasing its resilience and flexibility. This is precisely the modern definition of health. OPCs help the body to maintain its health in the best possible way.

The study was conducted over a period of eight

weeks with Masquelier's OPCs and a placebo in the control group. Its special feature was that it measured the physical condition of healthy people, namely male smokers. One of the results was that the OPCs group showed a significant improvement in vascular health. The total cholesterol and LDL cholesterol levels were significantly reduced and the antioxidant enzyme glutathione increased by 22 per cent, which meant an increase in immune defence. Anti-inflammatory effects increased with simultaneous stagnation of C-reactive protein and prostaglandin F2-alpha, among others. This study showed that OPCs maintain the cardiovascular homeostasis of smokers. This means that even smokers have a reduced risk of cardiovascular disease when taking OPCs. (Of course, this does not mean that OPCs make smoking completely harmless, as they have no effect on nicotine in cigarette smoke with its serious consequences for the lungs).

What you will find in this book: the physiological effect of OPCs

Based on the presentation of the French paradox, i.e. the contradiction between an unhealthy lifestyle in 20th century France and the simultaneously low risk of heart attacks among the red wine-loving French, **chapter I** provides you with information on red wine, alcohol and OPCs: What is the connection between wine consumption and the clumping of blood platelets? Why is red wine actually red? Why does it contain a lot of OPCs and white wine less? How many OPCs are contained in fruit?

In **chapter II**, we take a look at the history of seafaring: What does scurvy have to do with OPCs? Why were there ships in past centuries on which sailors fell victim to this terrible disease, while the crews of other ships were never affected? In this chapter you will also find a detailed list of OPCs applications, biochemical notes and practical information on the extraction of OPCs from plants, product quality, side effects and dosage. Exciting questions are answered: What does 'bio' actually mean? And how do we know that OPCs are 100 per cent 'bio', i.e. bioavailable? Why do OPCs increase the effect of vitamin C by a factor of ten? Are OPCs vitamin P? And what is a vitamin anyway?

Chapter III sheds light on the antioxidant effect of OPCs. Here you will learn how oxygen develops into dangerous free radicals, how these attack our cells throughout the body and thus cause various diseases. You will receive answers to the following questions: How do OPCs prevent our cells from becoming rancid? Why are they also known as anti-aging vitamins?

Chapter IV describes in detail the cholesterol cycle and its derailments as well as the mechanism by which OPCs prevent infarction in atherosclerosis and arteriosclerosis. In addition, the background to the strengthening and healing effects of OPCs in various areas is explained, such as improving thinking and concentration, poor eyesight, wounds and bone fractures, skin problems, hormonal disorders, headaches, inflammation and allergies. A large number of field reports illustrate the clinical studies cited.

Chapter V is dedicated to the aspect of beauty: How can you reduce wrinkles with OPCs and maintain smooth, fresh skin in the long term? Skin beauty is, of course, a mirror of the internal organs. The skin is the only organ that can also be viewed externally - and just as it can become wrinkled and scarred, so can all our internal organs and tissues that we cannot see. The condition of the skin reflects their condition in a certain way.

Finally, in **chapter VI** you will find information

on the equally impressive use of OPCs in animals. It is interesting to note that there is definitely no placebo effect in animals and that the purely physiological effect can be clearly observed here. In 1996, Professor Masquelier gave a lecture on OPCs in Baltimore, which left a strong impression in the USA and increased interest in this wonderful plant substance enormously. It is published in the **appendix**, along with a selection of scientific literature on the subject.

The breakthrough for OPCs is unstoppable

The scientific studies of the last 20 years read like a permanent confirmation of Professor Masquelier's discoveries in all their details. He was way ahead of his time. Jack Masquelier was as modest as he was brilliant. He observed nature with constant curiosity and sought to uncover its secrets. He succeeded - for the good of mankind. And yet he himself remained in the background and did not make a big fuss about himself. Nevertheless, it filled him with pride that the oligomeric procyanidins he discovered heal people as a frequently prescribed vascular protection drug in France and also protect against many diseases and premature aging worldwide. Preserving and giving health - few natural substances are able to do this as well as the OPCs isolated by Professor Masquelier. It is certainly no exaggeration to say that in another time and place his discoveries would have earned this great scientist the Nobel Prize. This did not happen, and so it is taking a little longer for OPCs to achieve the worldwide fame that this substance deserves - for the benefit of mankind. Its success is guaranteed, because OPCs are convincing in their own right, as they obviously bring people health and well-being.

Part I
The French Paradox:
Living Longer Through Red Wine

Regular red wine consumption prolongs your life

In 1979, the Welsh researcher A. S. St. Leger published an article in the renowned medical journal *The Lancet,* describing the connection between the mortality rate in industrialized countries and wine consumption. He came to the amazing conclusion that those countries did best where the most red wine was consumed - Italy and, ranking first, France. And this despite the fact that the French eat a fairly fatty diet and are heavy smokers. This paradox has come to be known as the 'French Paradox'.

Results achieved by the large-scale Copenhagen

study in 1995 were even more precise. In a comprehensive series of tests, Danish researchers concluded that regular wine consumption was the best protection against cardiac death and other fatal diseases. The risk of dying from a heart attack or stroke was reportedly reduced by sixty percent in the case of wine drinkers.

The French Paradox was also confirmed by a ten-year study called MONICA, which was commissioned by the World Health Organization to systematically compare the incidence of coronary heart disease on an international level starting in 1985. Countries such as France, Spain, Italy and Switzerland, where wine was consumed in relatively large quantities, showed the lowest mortality rate for coronary heart disease.

Is there an explanation for the French Paradox? Is alcohol genuinely healthy or is the decisive, relevant impact on our health due to other factors? As a matter of fact, alcohol as such has a 'blood-diluting' effect with beneficial consequences for the risk of infarction. It inhibits aggregation, i.e. the 'clotting' of blood platelets (thrombocytes) and thus reduces the likelihood of thrombosis. But this effect lasts only for a short period subsequent to alcohol intake. Then the so-called 'rebound effect' manifests itself, a reversal that occurs about 18 hours after alcohol consumption. The blood platelets become even more coagulable, resulting in an increased risk of blood clotting.

The only exception is red wine: although it is an alcoholic beverage, there is no danger of the rebound effect. On the contrary, when a moderate amount of red wine is regularly consumed, the blood contains less fibrinogen, the blood-clotting fibrous substances. Clots that have already formed are furthermore dissolved. This is an important factor in the prevention of heart attacks and strokes.

In contrast to other types of alcohol, the rebound effect does not manifest itself with red wine. What does red wine have that other alcoholic beverages don't?

It was not by chance that the French scientist Jack Masquelier finally succeeded in making the path-breaking discovery of these sought-after substances known as OPCs, which provide red wine with its health-supporting and life-prolonging properties. After all, Masquelier's homeland is the Bordelais, the region where the most delicious Bordeaux wines are produced.

OPCs are natural vegetable substances existing in a variety of fruit, in tree bark, skins and seeds, including grape seeds.

The history of the discovery of OPCs will be presented in more detail in the following chapter. Only this much shall be revealed at this point:

it proves how frequently major discoveries are based on chance. The discovery of OPCs, the substances that I will discuss here, however, has one peculiarity, which renders them hard for the researcher to detect: they are colourless.

Red wine contains considerable quantities of OPCs

Wine is made from grapes, whose skins and especially seeds, like other fruit, contain large quantities of OPCs. But why does only red wine contain OPCs and not white wine, which is made from grapes as well?

This mystery is solved when you compare the methods by which the two types of wine are produced. White wine is made from the juice of grapes. The grapes are pressed and the juice is collected and fermented until it turns into white wine. The seeds and skins are removed immediately after pressing.

In the case of red wine, on the other hand, the seeds and skins are fermented in the juice for a period of two to three weeks. During this time, the red pigments contained in the skins of the red grapes and the OPCs found primarily in the seeds can gradually dissolve in the wine. They lend the wine its red colour and enrich it with the substances that are responsible for the protective effect of red wine. Thus it becomes understandable why white wine is 20 to 50 times less rich in OPCs than red wine: in white wine, OPCs do not have the opportunity to pass from the seeds and skins into the juice, since they are discarded immediately after pressing.

The various protective effects of red wine can certainly be attributed to its phenolic substances, to OPCs. Moderate, regular consumption of red wine lowers the cholesterol level, has an antioxidant effect, stimulates the secretion of gastric juices, protects the teeth against caries, prevents inflammation, has an antibacterial effect, protects the heart and circulation and prolongs life.

Are those who do not drink any red wine condemned to malnutrition because they are likely to ingest insufficient quantities of OPCs?

Fortunately, this question can be negated, because a protected production method has been developed to harvest OPCs from pine bark and grape seeds. They are available in high concentration capsules or tablets.

Important Notice: The substance referred to in this book as OPCs exists in the same form in nature; it is produced in high concentration, through a patented process by Professor Masquelier. As there are less effective ways to obtain OPCs, I urgently advise you to acquire a product that conforms to the high quality standard according to Masquelier's patent. Research is based on this substance.

Multiple reactions:
Manfred K. 62, Poessneck[1]

I was always convinced that my diet was balanced and healthy. But then, ten years ago, I started taking OPCs (100 mg daily) as well as a compound of minerals, vitamins, and trace elements. My body's strong positive reaction revealed that I had obviously suffered from a deficiency before. I would never have thought it possible that these nutrients, which I have taken on an empty stomach every day since, could have such an extraordinarily favourable effect on my body.

Just three days after I started taking them, my bowel movements normalized. Now I hardly ever have flatulence. After about two weeks, I noticed I was physically much more able, especially in my sporting activities, like dancing, cycling, Nordic walking, swimming and winter sports. I hardly ever need my ten-minute afternoon nap, and I sleep well without waking up at night. As to my libido, I am going through my second adolescence. My blood values have improved considerably, bleeding stops

---

1   All case studies presented in this book have been carefully researched and documented. In all cases the affected persons ingested the OPCs preparation produced according to Masquelier's standards.

sooner although I am on blood thinners, and wounds heal faster now.

I am also free from pain now. Due to my profession - I am a master painter - I suffered from periods of pain in my right shoulder joint for over 15 years. An orthopaedist treated me with injections for the pain and an operation had already been planned. But now I am completely without pain. The pain caused by a slipped disc 22 years ago has also disappeared.

The food supplements have affected my appearance, too. I used to have lots of age spots, especially on the back of my hands, but also on my head and back. Now they have nearly completely disappeared.

My hair is more voluminous, and the wrinkles around my eyes and mouth are disappearing.

Finally, after taking OPCs for about four months, I am able to read the newspaper without glasses for the first time in 26 years, provided there is sufficient light. With my new vitality and agility, I am back to the weight and firm, flat stomach of my youth.

My quality of life is getting better and better all the time, so I take great pleasure in sharing my experience.

Part II
OPCs: The Discovery of a Wonderful Remedy

A glance back in history: rescue from death through scurvy

It is well known that in past centuries sailors were exposed to a major risk of contracting scurvy. For months they would be on the high seas. Their diet consisted of hard tack and salted meat since fresh fruit and vegetables were, of course, unavailable. But those who did not consume any fresh fruit or vegetables for more than two months either died or were terribly crippled.

Scurvy was the dreaded disease resulting from such a lifestyle. Malnutrition was the cause of bleeding gums and loss of teeth, changes in the bone structure, increased susceptibility to infection, haematoma, tissue destruction and, in the worst case, death from exhaustion. It is now known that the body's vitamin C reserves last about six weeks.

There are numerous examples from history confirming the mercilessness of an insufficient supply of vitamins. If the sailors deprived for months of fresh food were lucky, they ended up as hollow-eyed, toothless wrecks with crooked legs. When sailing around the Cape of Good Hope in 1498, Vasco da Gama lost almost two thirds of his crew to the fatal disease, which was more horrifying than the idea of shipwreck and a life and death struggle with stormy waves. This is the reason why sailors called it 'the gruesome disease'.

Another example of the destruction of the body due to vitamin C deficiency, in which a miraculous rescue occurred at the last moment, is the expedition of the French explorer Jack Cartier. His journey brought him and his crew of one hundred sailors to North America, today's Canada, in the winter of 1534/35. During several expeditions, he explored the St. Lawrence Bay, the Quebec area and sailed upriver into the interior of the country. He was surprised by a sudden cold spell. The river froze over trapping Cartier and his men to spend the entire winter there - a fatal situation for the crew. The logbook gives the details of this horrible winter: their gums receded to such an extent that they lost their teeth. Their breath was bad. The legs of some men became swollen, lost strength, turned black and failed them. Their skin turned blotchy. And finally they died. One corpse was dissected, since the helpless captain hoped to find the reason for the mysterious disease. They found a white, decomposing heart surrounded by red fluid ...

After 25 men had already died and another 15 were in critical condition, a native Indian came to their rescue. He directed Cartier to a tree, which he called 'Anneda', and explained how to concoct a tea from its bark and needles. The men who drank this liquid recovered within one week! They were recommended to put a poultice of the decoction on the afflicted body parts. In this way, the remaining crew managed to survive.

Cartier's encounter with the Indian shows that such life-saving measures in the struggle against the disease were a matter of luck. It took quite some time before vitamin deficiency was systematically diagnosed as the cause of the disorder. At least the benefits of oranges and lemons for the prevention of the deficiency disease were discovered in the 18th century by the British navy doctor James Lind. These could be taken on voyages. It was, however, only at the beginning of the 19th century that lemon juice became a regular daily component of the fare of British sailors. And only in the 20th century was it possible to isolate the ingredient of lemon juice responsible for preventing scurvy: anti-scurvy acid or rather ascorbic acid, today generally known as vitamin C.

On the track of vitamin C

In 1928, vitamin C was first isolated by the Hungarian scientist Albert Szent-Györgyi, who nine years later was awarded the Nobel Prize for this accomplishment. On closer scrutiny, ascorbic acid does not really deserve its name, since tests showed its pure synthetic form to be less effective against scurvy symptoms than the substance extracted from lemon peels ('citrin') or other raw materials such as peppers, which contain various ingredients in addition to vitamin C. One of life's ironies: Szent-Györgyi discovered vitamin C; but he actually spent his entire life looking for something different: OPCs. These colourless and thus long undiscovered substances are the co-factor of vitamin C, which the Nobel Prize winner never succeeded in identifying.[2]

---

2 In 1932, the American researchers W.A. Waugh and C.G. King called this substance, which they had also extracted from lemon juice, 'vitamin C'; in 1933, the Englishman

The discovery of OPCs

Professor Jack Masquelier's discovery of OPCs actually was a coincidental by-product of his doctoral thesis on the red pigment in peanuts. At the end of the Second World War, food was scarce and a lot of imagination was required to optimally utilize existing raw materials. Thus, Masquelier was assigned to determine whether the red skin surrounding the peanut underneath the shell contained any poisonous substances. The peanut residues, remaining after pressing peanut oil, were interesting both as animal fodder and for the starving people of the post-war period. Since some farmers complained that their cattle obviously did not like this fodder, it was necessary to find out about its potential toxicity.

Masquelier arrived at the conclusion that the red peanut skin did not contain any poisonous substances. In addition to the red substance, he identified other, colourless ingredients, which provided strong vascular protection: OPCs.

These OPCs obtained from peanut skin were applied to humans. The first test person was the pregnant wife of Masquelier's doctoral advisor, who suffered from oedema in her legs. An oedema is an accumulation of tissue fluid between the

H.C. Haworth and the Swiss T. Reichstein produced the first synthetic version.

cells due to an increased permeability of lymph and blood vessels. Only 48 hours after she had ingested the OPCs, the woman was cured - this provided the impetus for the intensive development of the first vasculo-protective medication based on OPCs. The drug was introduced to the French market in 1950 under the name 'Resivit'.

For better understanding:
OPCs - a few biochemical notes

- *Based on their pure chemical structure, OPCs could be categorized as flavonoids, but this classification is of little help since the range of this group of vegetal constituents is extremely broad. With respect to their biological utilization in the body and their level of toxicity and efficacy, the various flavonoids have highly diverging properties.*
- *Thus, Professor Masquelier suggested a new categorization. He wanted to place less emphasis on the rather meaningless group of flavonoids and instead concentrate on the group of flavanols.*
- *Oligomeric procyanidins are stable compounds of two, three, four and occasionally even five flavan-3-ol molecules, i.e. oligomeric (Greek: oligo = several) procyanidins: OPCs[3]. An individual flavan-3-ol*

3   The abbreviation OPCs has by now been generally accepted as technical term in many countries. In view of the rather complicated nomenclature of these molecule combinations, which furthermore differ in the English, Ger-

molecule is called a 'monomer'. If two of these molecules combine, they form a 'dimer', and three flavan-3-ol molecules constitute a 'trimer'.

- *Monomers on their own are not biologically active. But once they combine to form dimers and trimers, i.e. oligomers, they become effective. The term procyanidin refers to the fact that OPCs are colourless, but will turn red or blue under certain circumstances. Masquelier gave this group of substances its own name: pycnogenols.*

- *OPCs belong to the large group of vegetal substances known as polyphenols. This term comprises many different groups, including flavonoids and flavanols, which has resulted in considerable terminological confusion. OPCs have repeatedly been incorrectly referred to as flavonoids or bioflavonoids. They are, however, flavanols. For laymen, this differentiation may seem obscure, but it must be observed that the two groups have more differences than common features:*

- *Their only similarity is the flavane nucleus in their chemical structure. But otherwise, they differ in many respects: Flavonoids are not biologically active, whereas OPCs are 100% bioavailable, i.e. they can be completely used by the body. Some flavonoids have a toxic effect, whereas OPCs are*

man and French languages - ‚Procyanidols' or ‚Procyanidine' (French, German) and ‚proanthocyanidins' (English) - the term OPCs presents a simple solution which can be employed internationally.

completely harmless. In contrast to flavonoids, OPCs bond with proteins, especially collagen. Furthermore, flavonoids are yellow, whereas OPCs are colourless.

- *Thus, OPCs are highly specialized flavanols that are related but not equivalent to non-bioavailable tannins, which are contained in many foodstuffs such as vegetables, fruit juice, red wine, beer, cocoa, vinegar. The latter have an anti-viral effect, but remain in the digestive tract due to their molecular size. They do not enter into our blood circulation. This has been known for a long time, since tannins are effective remedies for diarrhoea.*

The significance of OPCs for humans

The range of OPCs' efficacy

1) Vessels

a) Legs
(extremities)

prophylaxis/ retardation/ treatment of:
- venous insufficiency
- starburst varices
- heavy legs
- venous congestion
- varicose veins
- varicose ulcers
- cold feet (and hands)
- chronic tingling sensation in legs
- 'formication'

b) Blood
circulation

regulation and strengthening of:
- cardiovascular system
- peripheral blood flow
- and prophylaxis for:
- high blood pressure

and prophylaxis for:
- stroke
- heart attack
- arteriosclerosis/atherosclerosis

c) Other vascular problems	*prophylaxis / retardation / treatment of:*
	• lymphatic congestion
	• haemorrhoids
	• thrombosis (aggregation)
	• sensitivity to changes in weather (permeability)
	• oedema
2. Allergies	*prophylaxis and treatment of:*
	• hay-fever (pollen, grass, trees)
	• allergy
	• asthma
3. Eyes	*prophylaxis / retardation / treatment of:*
	• cataracts
	• macula degeneration
	• decreasing vision
	• age-related sensitivity to light
	• night blindness
	• conjunctivitis
	• 'dry' eyes
	• glaucoma
4. Rheumatism, etc.	*prophylaxis / retardation / treatment of:*
	• arthritis
	• rheumatic disorders, in general
	• gout

5. Skin/collagen	*prophylaxis/retardation/treatment of::*
	• wrinkle formation
	• premature tissue wrinkles in organs
	• burns, sunburn
	• acne, eczema
	• neurodermatitis
	• psoriasis
	• cellulitis
	• stretch marks (pregnancy)
	Regulation and strengthening of:
	• skin elasticity
	• elasticity of toenails and fingernails
	• wound healing (acceleration)
	• dry skin
	• scar formation
	• collagen repair
6. Premature aging (antioxidant effects)	*prophylaxis/retardation/treatment of:*
	• Alzheimer's disease
	• Parkinson's disease
	• MS
	• senility
	• weak memory
7. Respiratory tract	*prophylaxis/retardation/treatment of:*
	• rhinitis (runny nose)
	• bronchitis
	• asthma
8. Injuries	*subsequent to injuries and surgery: detoxication and accelerated healing of:*
	• fractures, strains, tendons
	• muscular injuries, wounds in general

53

9. Diabetes	• strengthening of weakened tissue • revitalization in the case of fatigue
10. Blood lipids	• regulation of cholesterol
11. Female disorders	• PMS (premenstrual syndrome
12. CFS (Chronic Fatigue Syndrome)	• revitalizing and strengthening in the case of fatigue
13. Concentration	*(prophylactic) treatment of:* • hyperactivity, especially in children • learning disorders • concentration disorders in elderly people and children • reduced responsiveness, especially in elderly people
14. Vitamin booster	• increased efficacy of vitamins (A, C and E), minerals and trace elements
15. Immune system	*general boosting* • resistance toward flu and cold
16. Libido	*strengthening of:* • erectility • ability to reach orgasm

17. Inflammation *positive effect on all diseases ending in '-is' and '-itis', including*
- arthritis (joint inflammation)
- gastritis (inflammation of the gastric mucosa)
- hepatitis (liver inflammation)
- meningitis (inflammation of the brain membrane)
- periodontitis (gum inflammation)
- sinusitis (sinus inflammation)

This lengthy list confirms the importance of sufficient OPCs intake for our health, especially for blood and lymph vessels, eyes, general and psychic well-being and vitality as well as for the immune system.

How can the various effects of OPCs on the entire organism be explained?

- OPCs are strong antioxidants that effectively fight the dreaded free radicals and thus constitute a protective factor against cell damage. They can actually be described as the strongest antioxidants. Their antioxidant effect is 18 to 20 times stronger than that of vitamin C and 40 to 50 times stronger than that of vitamin E.
- OPCs regulate the cholesterol level in the blood.
- OPCs strengthen blood vessels and thus pre-

vent cardiovascular disorders. Since, in contrast to vitamin C, they bond with protein, particularly with collagen and elastin, they are able to double the resistance of blood and lymphatic vessels within 24 hours.

- OPCs improve blood circulation in the entire body and have a positive effect on vision, connective tissue, joints, mucous membranes, etc.
- Under the influence of OPCs, stress can be more easily tolerated.
- Memory is strengthened.
- Aging processes are slowed down: wrinkles form less rapidly, since the skin and underlying tissues remain supple and elastic longer.
- OPCs prevent caries.
- Arthritic inflammations as well as sports injuries heal more rapidly if OPCs are ingested.
- OPCs prevent allergic responses.

An impressive list, which makes the heart beat faster in view of the promising prospect of a long life in health and beauty!

Multiple allergies:
Manuela M., 29, Eschbach

Since I started working as a hairdresser at the age of 15, I have had multiple allergies, primarily to chemicals in cleaning agents, hair dye, perfumes, rubber, latex, etc. Various treatments, e.g. at the dermatological clinic of the University of Freiburg, didn't help. Cortisone injections and ointments were no use. I kept suffering from open wounds on my hands and arms. Since August 2004 I have taken OPCs (200 mg per day with a body weight of about 70 kg). I got better within four weeks. The open wounds closed and my skin has stopped itching.

Open leg ulcer, varicose veins:
Thomas H., 39, Allgaeu

For many years I suffered from an open leg ulcer that would not heal despite manifold treatments (traditional medicine, homeopathy, leeching and vitamin B12 injections). Because of this, two years ago my sister-in-law recommended OPCs and a combination of micronutrients which she herself had found helpful. I decided to try it and took 400 mg of OPCs plus micronutrients daily. For the first month it got worse and the wound discharged a lot of pus. To my relief, it started healing after that. I gradually lowered the dosage to 200 mg of OPCs daily.

However, I continued to suffer from bad varicose veins so that a light blow sufficed to injure my leg and open it up again. Even though these wounds healed very quickly, I decided in the end to have the varicose veins removed in an operation.

This turned out to be the right decision. After the operation I took 400 mg of OPCs daily, which accelerated the healing process. Now I am back to 200 mg. My leg has healed completely and is perfectly sound.

Stroke: Monika K., 60, Waibstadt

Four years ago, I had a stroke and my left side was paralyzed. For fourteen days I was completely immobile, incontinent, unable to speak, my sight was blurred, and I had bowel problems and trouble swallowing. In addition, tests showed I had hepatitis B. What bothered me the most, however, was that I was not able to understand a lot of things anymore.

I took various drugs for hypertension and diabetes and blood thinners. At the rehabilitation sanatorium I gradually improved due to water gymnastics and Reiki.

Although I slowly learnt to read texts again, I had difficulty in understanding their meaning. I tired quickly, but sleep brought no relief and my memory was bad. For a long time, I could not grasp things and could only walk on crutches. I also had trouble making myself understood, as I spoke slowly and swallowed syllables. I suffered from flatulence and had permanent bowel problems. Due to incontinence, I needed diapers.

The turning point came two and a half years later. In August 2005 I started taking OPCs (400 mg daily).

I noticed a quick improvement to my general condition. Five months later, I began to reduce my medication. Now I haven't taken anything for five months and yet my blood values have continually improved, especially the blood sugar levels.

Now all those troubles have nearly completely disappeared. I can walk without crutches again and even dance. My major problems have vanished. I can concentrate and remember things now. I have no problem understanding connections and I can articulate much better. I even have about 98 percent of my former strength in my right hand. Even if I occasionally have flatulence, I feel infinitely better and am happy. People can see this, for they keep telling me that I look much younger than last year. I feel like I have been given a second life.

'Healthy diet'?

The discussion about a healthy diet, which is now in all the media, makes us more and more aware of its importance for our health. But we find that industrial methods of production are frequently responsible for foodstuffs losing their vital nutrients during processing. Canned fruit is, for example, deprived of its peel. Even those who assume that consuming fresh fruit ensures an optimal provision with vital substances may err. It depends on the fruit. Only totally ripe fruit is replete with OPCs, while unripe fruit contains only very small quantities. Providing a whole society with fruit necessitates premature harvesting: transport, packaging, distribution and purchase by the final consumer take time. When buying fruit and vegetables, consumers should pay close attention to the degree of ripeness. Unripe fruit does not fulfil the expectations that diet-conscious consumers have for fresh food.

Our body does not produce OPCs or vitamin C itself. It is dependant on a regular intake of both substances. Now you may wonder why we cannot simply ingest OPCs with our regular diet, since they are contained in so many plants. The answer is simple: they are widely distributed in nature, but are mostly found in barks, shells, peels and woody parts which we tend to remove before we eat fruit. Thus, even people who set great store by a healthy diet can suffer a shortage of OPCs. The additional ingestion of OPCs to supplement our regular diet is therefore sensible. Moreover, OPCs are only found in tree or bush ripened fruit. In times of mass production, however, fruit is often picked before it is ripe and allowed to 'ripen' during transport. This prematurely harvested fruit contains hardly any OPCs.

OPCs extraction

The bark of the pine tree *Pinus maritima*, which is native to Les Landes, a region south of Bordeaux, contains huge quantities of the required substances. So OPCs were extracted from pine bark and processed into another vasoprotective medication called *Flavan*. In extracting OPCs from pine bark, Masquelier strove for an optimal ratio between raw material and obtained extract. During the extraction process, as high a concentration of OPCs as possible should be obtained from a given quantity of pine bark.

Due to the extremely high water solubility of OPCs, the ground bark is first dissolved in boiling water, a process closely resembling tea preparation. In addition to OPCs, other water-soluble substances dissolve. In order to obtain the highest possible concentration of OPCs, Masquelier developed a procedure whereby the proportion of OPCs and OPCs precursors ranged between 85 and 90 percent. Catechin, another substance, which is also water-soluble, is contained as well. But this is not a disadvantage. On the contrary, the presence of OPCs activates the catechins, thereby enabling their beneficial properties to develop. Thus, this process generates a highly potent flavanol mixture, the phytonutrient OPCs.

The preparations produced according to Professor Masquelier's patented process are unique in their efficacy since they guarantee an extremely high OPCs content as well as catechins and contain hardly any tannins, which are not bioavailable. In the case of products not manufactured according to the patented Masquelier method, the OPCs proportion may drop to a few percent and they may contain numerous substances that are not bioavailable (see 'Qualitative Features').

In 1955, Masquelier succeeded in proving that the identical OPCs molecules which he extracted from peanut skin and pine bark are also contained in red wine - and that these flavanols by far exceed flavonoids, such as rutin, with respect to their vasoprotective properties.

Now the question is where else flavanols exist in nature. Answer: in many plants which we consume every day, such as fruits and vegetables, and in those whose healing properties we already know in other contexts, such as *ginkgo biloba*, mistletoe, hawthorn, as well as in the bark of certain trees, such as the Australian tea tree, as was illustrated in the historical examples previously described.

The mysterious rescue of Cartier's crew through the bark and needles of the Anneda tree can today be easily explained by Masquelier's insights. The bark of the Anneda tree is obviously rich in OPCs, while the needles contain high amounts of vitamin C. Thanks to this unbeatable team, the sailors obtained an effective remedy, which saved their lives despite their extremely poor physical condition.

In the industrial extraction of a natural substance, the ratio between expenditure and yield is decisive. Masquelier focused on the production of OPCs from pine bark and grape seeds, since they have a tremendously high concentration of OPCs and, furthermore, are so-called 'by-products'. Pines are not felled for the production of OPCs, but in order to manufacture paper and to obtain timber. Thus, the bark is 'left', as are grape seeds, which are a by-product of juice and wine production.

Qualitative features

OPCs are predominantly taken from the bark of *Pinus maritima* and primarily from the grape seeds of *Vitis vinifera,* but it would be wrong to equate OPCs with pine bark or grape seed extracts. Vitamin C is not equivalent to orange juice and OPCs are not identical with grape seed extract. The latter term can be applied to any substance gained from grape seeds, whereby the OPCs content may be minimal. Like vitamin C, which is obtained according to standardized methods of production, OPCs are pure substances that can be gained from pine bark and grape seed as well as from many other plants.

In the USA 'grape seed extract' headed the list of dietary supplements in 1996, 1997 and 1998. But unfortunately, this is not only good; they should have been more precise. Every successful natural remedy attracts countless charlatans and crooks, and this applies particularly to OPCs products.

In 1997, an independent laboratory in Chelmsford, Massachusetts, examined the antioxidant properties of three grape seed and pine bark products produced according to Masquelier's method, as well as ten other 'grape seed extracts' sold on the U.S. market.

The result: the three preparations which were produced according to Masquelier's patented process contained at least 85 percent OPCs and their components (i.e. active substances) and turned out to be potent and biologically effective remedies. This patented OPCs product is the only preparation where OPCs have been scientifically studied over many years. 'Masquelier's OPCs' have been tested according to strict guidelines, have been deemed beneficial, have been patented (in various countries) and have even been recognized as medical ingredients in pharmaceutical products in France. There they still are, more than 50 years after their discovery, the active substances most frequently prescribed for the treatment of vascular fragility.

In the independent laboratory test in Chelmsford mentioned above, the other grape seed extracts - with one exception - all had rather poor results. Some did not contain any OPCs whatsoever, others only a minimal amount.

OPCs' bioavailability to the body

In order to be recognized as a medication, a substance is subject to extremely strict and comprehensive controls and must fulfil a number of criteria, including 'bioavailability'. What is bioavailability?

The vital ingredients which we ingest with food are resorbed in the various sections of our digestive system, i.e. they pass the barrier of gastric and intestinal walls and are then absorbed by the blood vessels and transported to all parts of the body.

This process happens in varying degrees. Some substances are resorbed only poorly, others not at all, which means that they are not available to the body as nutrients.

A substance which is ingested but is then discharged from the digestive tract is of hardly any use to the body. It is not bioavailable. Thus, we can obviously only benefit from the miraculous properties of a substance if our body can actually use it.

How can the bioavailability of a substance be determined? Proof of OPCs' bioavailability was furnished by means of radioactivity. Vines cultivated in the laboratory were exposed to minuscule concentrations of radioactivity. Their grape seeds were processed into OPCs extract and orally administered to laboratory animals - rats, mice and guinea pigs. After a certain period of time an x-ray revealed that the OPCs had spread throughout the entire body: from the intestines they had passed into the blood stream and could be traced in all tissues, including skin, hair, nails as well as various organs. This meant optimal bioavailability of the OPCs substance that had been dissolved in water. An especially high concentration of OPCs could be detected in the aorta, the walls of the duodenum, liver, bronchial tubes and skin, as well as in the cartilage of the sternum, spleen, glands, lungs, plasma, cardiac muscle, muscles and blood. OPCs immediately pass into the blood stream. Only ten minutes after ingestion, OPCs could already be detected in the blood of the laboratory animals. The rapid availability of a substance is, of course, of particular importance in emergencies, such as allergic attacks. The highest concentration was reached after 45 minutes, and then the level gradually dropped. After seven hours, it still ranged at about one third of the maximum level. OPCs are discharged to a small degree (14 percent after eleven hours) via the bile, i.e. via the intestines.

OPCs and vitamin C - an unbeatable team

The importance of vitamin C for a well-functioning organism has already been discussed. It influences almost all our metabolic processes. In contrast to most animals, humans are unfortunately not able to produce this indispensable vitamin themselves. They must ingest it with food. Linus Pauling, the great vitamin C researcher, examined how much ascorbic acid is produced by animals and then deduced the quantity of ascorbic acid required by humans, depending on age, weight and size. He arrived at a significant maximum of 18 g per day, a dosage that considerably exceeds general guidelines. Normally a daily quantity of about 100 mg is recommended.

With his book on vitamin C published in 1970, Linus Pauling, who was awarded the Nobel Prize twice, triggered a vitamin C boom. From then on many people followed the megadoses that he recommended and expected a life-prolonging, cell-rejuvenating and resistance-boosting effect - and quite rightly so. Pauling himself, who took 12 g of vitamin C daily, was a very healthy man until his death at the ripe old age of 93 years. Small wonder in view of the incredible protective functions that this vitamin carries out for the organism!

Protective properties of vitamin C

- It is indispensable for growth, especially for the formation of collagen, which is contained in bones, cartilage, skin, tendons, sinews and tissue as scleroprotein. It safeguards the elasticity and health of said structures and provides protection from infections.
- Ascorbic acid is a tremendously effective antioxidant which prevents the dangerous free radicals (see further on) from destroying body cells. It also saves other vitamins, such as certain B-vitamins, vitamin A and E, from oxidation.
- Vitamin C is involved in the production and/or activation of red blood cells, defence cells, folic acid and hormones.
- Vitamin C absorbs carcinogenic nitrates and

nitrites and thus performs an anti-carcino-
genic function.
- It is responsible for transporting iron in the
blood and providing sufficient oxygen for the
cells.
- Vitamin C is indispensable for healing wounds
and maintaining healthy blood vessels.

What Pauling did not know: he might have been
able to reduce the dosage of vitamin C and at
the same time achieve an even higher efficacy for
his body, since OPCs are substances that greatly
boost the effect of vitamin C.

Let us refresh our memories: Albert Szent-Györgyi, the Hungarian discoverer of vitamin C, was
actually searching for the co-factor of vitamin C.
Research had shown that pure synthesized vitamin C was less effective in fighting scurvy than
vegetal extracts, e.g. from lemon peels, which
contain other substances in addition to vitamin
C. Thus, he assumed that one of these substances
supported vitamin C and that the combination
of the two would have a particular healing effect.
He was, however, not able to determine which
substance it was.

This evidence was finally furnished in 1976 by
Masquelier and his colleagues within the frame-
work of a path-breaking study. In various contexts, it had become obvious that OPCs multi-

plied the effect of vitamin C. One example was the lowering of the cholesterol level by OPCs, an effect that was significantly increased by the intake of vitamin C. How could the assumption that OPCs were the sought-after co-factor of vitamin C be corroborated? Masquelier performed an experiment with guinea pigs, which was as simple as it was impressive. These animals belong - like primates and some kinds of bats - to the few species that are not able to synthesize vitamin C and - like humans - are dependant on ingesting a sufficient amount through their food.

An impressive experiment: The guinea pigs were divided into five different lots and furnished with varying quantities of vitamin C. The higher the daily dosage of vitamin C, the more vigorous the animals were and the longer they lived. The amazing result of this examination was that animals that were given a low quantity of vitamin C, i.e. 5 mg per kilo of body weight per day, as well as an additional dosage of OPCs were in as good a condition as those that had been provided with a sufficient quantity of vitamin C, that is 20 mg of vitamin C per kilo of body weight per day.

Thus, OPCs act as a vitamin C booster, which ensures survival even if the body is not provided with enough vitamin C. As a matter of fact, the amount of vitamin C required drops to one tenth under the effect of OPCs.

According to this calculation, Linus Pauling would have needed only 1.2 g of ascorbic acid instead of his daily dosage of 12 g if he had supplemented it with OPCs, and would still have enjoyed excellent health and vitality as he got older. Now the question arises which substance supports the other: do OPCs boost vitamin C or vice versa? This question can be answered quite easily. Both substances enhance one another. By administering vitamin C, the remedial properties of OPCs are intensified, while the beneficial properties of vitamin C are multiplied by OPCs. In both cases, healing processes are initiated and/or accelerated. In combination, OPCs and vitamin C are an unbeatable team!

Are OPCs vitamin P?

Let us remember the example of the wife of Masquelier's doctoral advisor whose oedema healed within two days after ingesting OPCs. Or, looking even further back, think of the dreaded scurvy, which Cartier's crew narrowly escaped, thanks to the Anneda tree. The typical symptoms of scurvy include the disintegration of the body's tissue if no fresh fruit and vegetables have been eaten over an extended period of time. As it was impossible to refrigerate certain foods or preserve their freshness in any other way, seafarers took dried meat, cereal and, of course, liquor on their voyages. In the 18th century, the situation improved for British sailors when a navy doctor discovered the connection between citrus fruit and scurvy prevention. But it was only in the last century that the discovery of vitamin C revealed the reason for this connection.

Vitamins are organic compounds required by the body in order to sustain vital processes. Since vitamins (with the exception of vitamin K and, by daylight, also vitamin D) are not produced by the body itself, we have to ingest them via our food. The lack of certain vitamins in the body results in deficiency symptoms.

Some vitamins can be stored in the body over a fairly long period, but eventually these deposits are depleted unless we replenish them with appropriate vitamins from our food. Regular vitamin intake from outside is indispensable.

Possibilities for storing vitamins:

- B12: up to five years
- A: up to two years
- E: six to twelve months
- D and folic acid: two to four months
- C, B2 and K: two to six weeks

- B1: maximum of two weeks
- OPCs: 72 hours

Some experts regard OPCs as a vitamin, specifically vitamin P, which is responsible for the permeability of the capillaries, the extremely fine branches of the blood and lymphatic vessel system. Thus, the following statement can be found in a scientific study published by the pharmaceutical faculty of Bordeaux University: 'Flavanol oligomers are practically the only source of vitamin P in our food. [...] They are easily soluble, completely bioavailable, non-toxic, non-mutagenic [i.e. they do not cause any hereditary changes in the genetic material] and non-carcinogenic [not cancer producing]. They [...] have a justified claim to vitamin status.'[4]

Vitamin P is responsible for reducing capillary permeability. In addition, it has inflammation-inhibiting and anti-allergic properties.

---

4 J. Masquelier, J. Michaud, K. Bronnum-Hansen, Faculté de Pharmacie, Bordeaux: 'Recherche et dosage des Oligomères Flavanoliques dans les Aliments d'Origine Végétale'; quoted in Bert Schwitters: OPCs in Action. Rome 1997 (2nd edition), p. 56.

When is a vitamin a vitamin?

A vitamin is defined as a non-mineral compound minute quantities of which are vital for the organism. The body cannot produce this substance itself, so that it must be supplied through food. After a certain period, the lack or insufficient supply of a vitamin results in known deficiency symptoms: a vitamin C deficiency is responsible for scurvy; a vitamin D deficiency causes rickets; the lack of certain B vitamins produces beriberi etc. Allergies, susceptibility to infection, digestive problems, lack of concentration and many other disorders can frequently be attributed to a deficiency of vital substances.

In this respect, the discovery of vitamin C was a major achievement, for which Szent-Györgyi certainly deserved the Nobel Prize. However, as already mentioned, tests showed that pure synthetically-produced ascorbic acid was less effective in fighting scurvy than when the substance was ingested in the form of fruit, where it is combined with other substances. 'Citrin', a mixture of substances extracted from lemon peels, is a more potent vaso-protector than pure vitamin C. Because of its effect on vascular permeability, the scientist called citrin 'vitamin P'.

A substance is granted the status of a vitamin only when evidence can be furnished that the lack of it results in deficiency symptoms in the body. This was never proven by Szent-Györgyi. As a matter of fact, it is very probable that OPCs are the sought-after vitamin P and were just not noticed due to their small size and lack of colour.

Open wounds, connective tissue, varicose veins: Lisbeth W., 47, France

For some months I've been taking OPCs every day and have had good experience with it. For several years again and again I had open wounds on the groin and horrible itching. After I started taking 2 x 100 mg OPCs/day the wound healed within a week and the itching was gone. I used to have cracks on my fingers and heels, but since taking OPCs this has stopped. On the whole, my skin has become supple and soft. Since my problems went away, I've been taking 100 mg per day.

My connective tissue has tightened a lot. I've had six children, therefore a 'wobbly' stomach, and I weighed ten kilograms more than before my pregnancies. Within four months I've lost four kilos and my stomach has become firm. I don't have cravings since I started taking OPCs together with a vitamin mineral compound. Even my vagina has tightened a lot. My husband says that I'm like a virgin.

I don't feel my varicose veins anymore.

OPCs - protection for all blood and lymph vessels

OPCs are substances that protect blood and lymph vessels. How do they manage to do this?

Since OPCs can bond with proteins, they attach to collagen and elastin, components of the vascular wall. Both are so-called scleroproteins of the connective tissue. Collagen is, moreover, present in sinews, cartilage and bones. The task of collagen and elastin is to build vascular walls and keep them strong and supple. By attaching to these two proteins - which vitamin C is not able to do - OPCs activate their synthesis and metabolism and prevent their premature decay.

Many people know the term 'collagen' from cosmetic products that promise skin regeneration and smoothness through application of creams containing collagen. As two essential constituents of the vascular wall, collagen and elastin ensure its elasticity and permeability. Collagen can be thought of as a type of track with regular crosslinks or as a ladder with rungs connecting the two supports. The lateral parts consist of protein chains, polypeptides that are intertwined. Of great importance for the stability and elasticity of these chains is the number of rungs if we want to stay with the simile of the ladder. If they break, the connective tissue becomes weak and permeable. At the spots where rungs have broken, there are gaps where blood and lymphatic fluid leak into the surrounding tissue, resulting in haematoma, oedema and dropsy.

But the opposite is not desirable either. Under the influence of free radicals, crossed rungs develop, which make the connective tissue rigid, resulting in premature wrinkles. This development, however, is regulated by OPCs, which are potent antioxidants and thus effective scavengers of free radicals.

This is why Professor Masquelier regards OPCs as the vitamin of the vascular wall - vitamin P.

Weak bladder: Alexa B., 51, Sulz a/N.

After giving birth to my daughter, I suffered from a weak bladder, which despite regular pelvic floor exercises grew worse and worse. Twenty years later I had come to the point where I could not move anymore without being afraid of 'accidents'. I was therefore willing to have an operation on my urethra. Thanks to a friend who advised me against such an operation because of the numerous complications, I postponed it for a while - until I finally realized that the problem no longer existed. In the meantime, I had started taking OPCs (a daily dose of 200 mg with a body weight of 50 kg). I am convinced that taking OPCs regularly freed me from my bladder trouble.

How do you know that your vascular walls are weakened?

- If your gums bleed when you brush your teeth,
- if hardly noticeable pressure, pinching or nipping results in haematoma,
- if you are terribly tired in the evenings although your day has not been that strenuous,
- if you frequently notice some blood in your cornea,
- if water tends to accumulate in your legs and arms in warm weather or
- if your legs feel tired and swollen in the evenings,

you probably suffer from weakened or hypersensitive vascular walls, which can be strengthened by taking OPCs.

Sense of smell, skin, spider veins, cellulitis: Claudia H., 46, Verl

For six months I've 'enjoyed' OPCs enthusiastically! Thanks to this high quality antioxidant (200 mg daily with a body weight of 59 kg) I have regained my sense of smell. For two years I wasn't able to smell or taste anything between 9 pm and 9 am (and sometimes even longer). My skin has improved considerably, and I've also noticed other improvements in many little things, i.e. fewer spider veins and less cellulitis. I was absolutely

*amazed and overjoyed to realize that a tiny wart that I
had had for many years wasn't there anymore.*

*The decrease in my spider veins has made me aware
that also all the other, invisible vessels in my body are
strengthened and protected. This 'inner care' makes me
feel good and secure regarding my future health. As a
preventologist I've studied healthy diets and diet supplementation and I am very grateful to have found out
about OPCs.*

Application, side effects and dosage

In the many years of scientific research on OPCs,
no side effects have been detected. OPCs are not
poisonous, but healing and beneficial in many respects. They are a remedy that maintains or restores health. Thus, they can be used both as a
medication and as a dietary supplement to prevent disease. Studies performed by the Pasteur
Institute confirm that OPCs are not toxic, not
carcinogenic (cancer producing) and not muta-
genic (altering the genetic material). Long-term
ingestion of a dosage of 35,000 mg (!) per day
over a period of six months did not result in any
negative consequences to the organism.

Nevertheless, one aspect should be mentioned:
Since OPCs activate the vitamin C supplies in the

body and harmonize blood flow, they may occasionally result in an increased excretion of toxic substances deposited in the organism (heavy metals, herbicides, pesticides, etc.). This process may cause an initial feeling of indisposition, which will, however, disappear after about a week and is usually followed by a noticeable increase in vitality.

Recommended dosages

- *If OPCs are taken as a dietary supplement in order to maintain health and well-being, the recommended daily dosages range from 1 to 2 mg per 1 kg of body weight. Thus, a person weighing 50 kg should take 50 to 100 mg per day. In stressful situations, the quantity can be doubled.*

- *If OPCs are used as a therapy for certain health problems, the dosage may be significantly higher. Scientific literature reports studies where up to 500 mg were administered per day without any noticeable interaction with other drugs or side effects. These dosages were administered in the treatment of varicose legs, retinopathy, PMS, sports injuries and post-surgical oedema.*

Some facts about OPCs

- Within minutes OPCs are absorbed into the blood through the oral and gastric mucosa and transported to all body tissues.
- After a few minutes, they can already be detected in the blood.
- They are 100% bioavailable.
- They are water-soluble.
- They reach their highest concentration in the blood after about 45 minutes. They are completely used up in the body within 72 hours.
- Due to their small molecular size, OPCs - like vitamin C - pass the blood, brain and spinal cord barrier and unfold their remedial properties also in regions that are not reached by most other substances.
- The resistance of blood vessels doubles already 24 hours after ingesting OPCs.

From a chemical and biological viewpoint, OPCs are clearly of major importance for the human organism. The body cannot produce these substances itself but requires them to sustain vital functions. We have seen that there are good arguments for regarding OPCs as a vitamin, and that their vital substances are indispensable for vascular health. The list of deficiency diseases resulting from lack of OPCs is long and alarming.

Periodontosis with jawbone degeneration:
Anne L., 42, Munich

Around my 40th birthday, I experienced a health crisis which manifested itself primarily in a dramatic recession of my gums and jawbone degeneration. Although I was afraid of losing all of my teeth within a few years, I underwent complete dental restoration and had all amalgam fillings replaced by gold crowns. Tests showed that I had high concentrations of mercury in my body. In addition, I also underwent jaw surgery, so-called 'open curettage', and was fastidious in oral hygiene. Despite all these efforts, it was hard to maintain a healthy state, I frequently responded to stress with painful gum inflammation and noticeable gum recession.

After I had started taking OPCs, I gradually began to feel better. The condition of my gums stabilised. And then an x-ray that my dentist took of two teeth revealed an amazing fact: the bone, which had already half-degenerated, was again clearly visible on the x-ray. Five of us compared old x-rays with the new one: There was no doubt that my jawbone had regenerated in this spot. My dentist could not explain this phenomenon; we had already discussed the option of implanting bone from my hip in the jaw ...

Part III
OPCs for a Long Life in Good Health

Free radicals - a modern danger

Only a few years ago, nobody could expect laypersons to be familiar with the term 'antioxidant'. But this no longer holds true. Our society has become much more conscious of health issues in the meantime. This is in direct response to a more strenuous lifestyle in general, with increasing physical and psychic strain. Immune diseases are on the rise. A primary cause for this development is the fact that our bodies are no longer able to balance the positive and negative aspects of oxidation processes.

The term oxidation refers to the process of oxygen bonding with a different chemical element.

We know many natural oxidation processes: if iron corrodes or butter turns rancid, this is the result of oxygen reactions. And we also owe the visible biological aging of our body to oxygen.

Oxygen, however, performs not only destructive but also life-giving functions. Masquelier calls oxygen 'a Janus-faced person, somebody with a good as well as a very dangerous side'. We could also say: oxygen is like Dr. Jekyll and Mr. Hyde.

Oxygen means life: we need oxygen to breathe. Oxygen is also required for a functioning metabolism. Here it assumes the task of splitting nutrients, which the body uses for energy, growth and regeneration. Oxygen molecules have other beneficial effects: they play a major part in the body's own immune system and defend our organism against certain bacteria and other intruders. In the latter case, our immune system avails itself of the toxicity of oxygen. So much for the Dr. Jekyll feature.

By now, though, oxygen has become more famous for its appearance in the shape of the dangerous, unpredictable Mr. Hyde: oxygen radicals are not stable. They either have one electron too many or one too few, and thus, in a 'radical' manner, constantly try to connect with other substances in order to regain stability. These oxygen radicals, that are highly reactive due to the instability, have achieved notoriety. In practice, antioxidants are their counterparts. As a matter of fact, radical oxygen molecules - referred to as 'free radicals' - are considered to be the most dangerous attackers of our immune system and are held responsible for a multitude of chronic diseases, including cancer, cardiovascular disorders, allergies, cataracts and many more. They incapacitate the body's natural defence systems. But they succeed in doing so only after a certain period. In youth, the body's own protective systems usually suffice, but after a certain age they disintegrate. Chronic problems with wear and tear and exhaustion usually manifest themselves after the age of 40, when the free radicals in the body no longer encounter any resistance, thus enabling them to perform their destructive attack on body tissue and blood vessels uninhibited.

Medical and scientific experts increasingly focus on the danger emanating from free radicals in the genesis of numerous diseases. By now free radicals are considered the primary culprits responsible for the aging process. They contribute to the development of certain diseases including arteriosclerosis, rheumatism, diabetes, allergies, Parkinson's disease, immune deficiencies and high blood pressure. What exactly are free radicals?

They are molecular biochemical substances in human body cells. They have either one electron too many or one too few, so that they are constantly trying to combine with other substances in order to balance the missing or excess electron. This constant reaction in the cells is only beneficial if the defence cells of the immune system are stimulated to fight pathogenic organisms. Another positive effect of free radicals is the release of energy when oxygen combines with other chemical substances.

But if there are too many free radicals in the body cells, oxidation processes take place, which aggressively attack our cells. The cells' own fatty substances turn 'rancid' and the previously mentioned disorders quickly manifest themselves.

Free radicals have their origin in cigarette smoke, x-rays, the sun's UV radiation, nitrite and nitrate residues in food and in the body cells, where oxygen is incompletely converted. The body checks free radicals by means of enzymes. But these are powerless in the presence of an excessive number of radicals.

It is then that the body requires help from outside: the so-called antioxidants, substances which counteract the oxidation process. They include primarily enzymes, the vitamins C, E and beta carotene, selenium - and above all: OPCs!

Why have free radicals suddenly assumed such an important and dangerous role for our organism? What has changed about our lives? The sad answer is that we humans are ourselves largely responsible for the predominance of this dangerous potential. In addition to natural oxidation, stress and environmental toxins trigger artificially induced oxidative responses.

Environmental toxins: Through the air that we breathe and the water we drink we are exposed to ten thousands of different chemical poisons, ranging from cigarette smoke, exhaust fumes and detergent emissions to numerous chemical additives including preservatives, flavour enhancers, colorants, synthetic sweeteners and all the other ingredients contained in pre-cooked meals, sauce and soup concentrates and many other 'foodstuffs'. Insecticides (lindane, DDT), pesticides, fungicides, fertilizers (nitrate, nitrite) and numerous chemical substances (solvents and halogenated hydrocarbons, such as dioxin, PCP, PCB) as well as heavy metals (e.g. mercury in amalgam fillings) put tremendous strain on our immune system and support the position of Mr. Hyde.

Radiation: Excessive exposure to the sun, radioactivity, i.e. earth radiation, as well as the low and high frequency rays emitted by numerous state-of-the-art devices, expose the body to excessive radiation resulting in intense oxidation processes.

Stress: Free radicals are closely linked to stress. They generate stress and conversely are a result of stress. An individual suffering from stress is in a poor physical condition. The weakened organism is unable to protect itself against the attack of free radicals. Conversely, they cause oxidative stress in the body, especially in the case of Aids, and thus, a vicious cycle is set in motion.

Free radicals damage, injure, alter:
- cell membranes
- DNA and genes
- fats and proteins
- cells

Free radicals accelerate:
- disintegration of tissue and thus
- aging processes

Free radicals are responsible for an accelerated course of certain degenerative disorders, such as:
- respiratory disorders
- arteriosclerosis
- cancer
- vascular disorders
- diabetes
- mucoviscidosis
- hepatitis
- inflammations
- organic brain disorders
- kidney failure
- rheumatic arthritis
- Alzheimer's disease
- Parkinson's disease

OPCs - the strongest antioxidants presently known

After this threatening list, we are coming to the positive part of this chapter: We do not have to helplessly and hopelessly surrender to free radicals. Fortunately, nature provides us with a number of protective agents, among which the antioxidants in our diet play an essential role. As natural antagonists to free radicals, they protect the body from oxygen-induced harm and can repair damage that has already developed.

The most important antioxidants include vitamin C (ascorbic acid), selenium, beta-carotene, vitamin E (tocopherol) and above all OPCs. We obtain these substances primarily from our food. This is also the reason why a healthy diet comprising plenty of seeds, vegetables and fruit from largely untreated, controlled biological cultivation is of utmost importance. The main suppliers of antioxidants are cereals, beans, meat, seafood and dairy products. Due to increasing environmental pollution, our body has to fight a rising number of free radicals, resulting in a soaring need for antioxidants.

What all antioxidants have in common is that they defend the organism against intruding oxygen radicals; but they have additional protective functions. Vitamin C boosts the immune system, vitamin E strengthens the heart, polyphenols (e.g. in green tea) help prevent cancer and beta-carotene protects the skin.

Among all these potent agents, some substances are particularly effective: OPCs. They combine a number of special benefits, giving them prominence over the other substances.

The special position of OPCs among antioxidants

- OPCs are quickly absorbed by the body and distributed all over the organism. They fight free radicals especially fast and limit their destructive potential. Thus they provide efficient protection against age-related symptoms of decay.
- OPCs scavenge free radicals all over the body.
- OPCs neutralize many different types of free radicals. They serve as efficient antioxidants both in fat as well as in water phases. This is where they differ from all other antioxidants, which become active either in a fatty or in an aqueous environment.
- OPCs neutralize free radicals in the body to a much greater extent than vitamin C and simultaneously enhance the effect of vitamin C.
- OPCs are also 40 to 50 times more effective

than vitamin E since they fight more (different) free radicals.
- This versatility makes OPCs the strongest 'radical scavengers', a match for all challengers.

Specialist for the connective tissue

Nevertheless, OPCs are particularly effective in one field. They protect connective tissue (especially collagen) against the assault of free radicals. Their long-term attack on the cell membranes of the body and immune cells results in alterations in the cellular walls. OPCs prevent the destruction of vascular membranes in the stomach, intestines, brain, respiratory tracts, joints and spine. Thus, they are able to check, or even reverse, degenerative disorders in these areas.

As antioxidants, OPCs remain unsurpassed thus far, especially since they have not only been tested in laboratory test tubes - *in vitro* -, but also extensively on living beings, that is *in vivo*.

In 1985, Masquelier furnished evidence that pure OPCs obtained from grape seeds and pine bark are by far more effective compared to other substances with known antioxidant properties, such as various bioflavonoids and vitamin C. Compared to the latter, OPCs were 18.4 times more powerful. Considering the fact that the antioxidant effect of vitamin C has been generally acknowledged, substances which are almost 20 times more potent provide reason for euphoria!

Furthermore, Japanese research results, independent of Masquelier's studies, were published almost at the same time and arrived at the identical conclusion: according to these studies, the antioxidant efficacy of OPCs is 40 to 50 times more powerful than that of vitamin E![5]

The thrilling discovery of the most potent natural scavengers of free radicals resulted in the registration of OPCs as a U.S. patent.

In 1987, OPCs were patented as antioxidants, substances which scavenge dangerous free radicals. Although it took a long time before OPCs were publicly acknowledged as the most important antioxidants, this area of activity was only logical: the protective ingredients which Masquelier had first discovered in the red skin surrounding the peanut, obviously prevented the oily substances contained in the nut from turning rancid. The same is true for pine bark, which prevents oxidation, or for the thin layer around the grape seeds and their oily insides. Since OPCs exist primarily in areas where easily oxidizable substances

5 Ushida, Edamatsu et. al.: 'Condensed tannins scavenge active oxygen free radicals', in: Med. Sci. Res. (15) 1987, pp. 831f.

require protection, one can clearly assume that they possess antioxidant properties.

The abstract describing the patent states, among other things, that 'the invention provides a method for preventing and fighting the harmful biological effects of free radicals in the bodies of warm-blooded animals and more especially in human beings, namely cerebral involution, hypoxia following arteriosclerosis, cardiac or cerebral infarction, tumour promotion, inflammation, ischemia, alterations of the synovial liquid, collagen degradation, among others.'[6]

Why OPCs are effective in treating the most varied diseases

That a single substance can be so broadly applied is normally an indication of minor efficacy. In the case of OPCs, however, a highly plausible explanation for their beneficial effect in the therapy of a variety of disorders exists. All of these diseases are attributable to an identical cause: an undue assault of free radicals on the body. Since they are active everywhere in the body, free radicals attack all cells, especially the fatty portions of cell membranes. An excessive oxygen attack on our

6   Cited according to Schwitters, loc.cit., p. 131

body cells causes us to gradually 'turn rancid':
Our immune system is no longer able to ward
off the assault, and we develop different diseases
in different places.

Masquelier impressively presents this process in
the following manner: 'You could say that for our
cells, aging is equivalent to turning rancid. Thus,
every cell suffers from the excessive oxidative effect of free radicals. And therefore, if cellular de-
composition in one or the other organ causes disease - or in yet another organ or another place: in
the teeth, the eyes, the brain, in the fingers, feet,
arteries etc. -, then some common factor must be
present which is fought by OPCs. OPCs do not
counteract 10,000 different free radicals. They
scavenge oxygen radicals, which are active in a
variety of living cells. If such cells are destroyed
- be it in the kidneys, the eyes or the heart -, such
destruction is the result of free radical activity.'

OPCs: an anti-aging vitamin

What are the ramifications of this discovery of
tremendously powerful antioxidants? Why make
such a fuss about effective scavengers of free radicals? Isn't this more a technical discussion, which
may be of some interest for biochemists, but is

of minor significance for ordinary people? Possibly. But it affects us all, whether we want it or not. Free radicals are responsible for our aging at a faster or a slower rate, they determine whether we fall ill earlier or later, whether we suffer from severe or minor disorders. With the help of potent antioxidants we can significantly and actively influence this struggle in our favour.

We cannot stop our aging process, since this biological development has been genetically programmed. But we can delay it and prevent the damaging side effects triggered by free radicals. In this respect, OPCs are certainly a serious anti-aging vitamin.

Can OPCs prolong our lives?

In many areas, the scientific research of OPCs has produced results that have been confirmed by a multitude of studies, but not with respect to 'life expectancy'. The question whether OPCs are able to prolong human life has yet to be answered.

In a few decades, there might be an unambiguous, positive reply if the appropriate test series were to be initiated now. Unfortunately, no definite statement can be made at this point. Still, sufficient animal experiments have been conducted, which have produced amazing results.

Some mammals have a relatively short life span so that we already have some results. Mice, for example, live for one to two years only. Tests have confirmed that OPCs increase this life expectancy by 30 to 40 percent.

Such experiments show that we can prolong life if we fight excessive cell oxidation. And the results of animal experiments may, to a certain degree, suggest that these apply to humans as well. It would, of course, be unrealistic to hope that our life expectancy could be doubled or tripled; but human DNA allows the possibility of 120 years of life. This period is shortened only by the unimpeded or insufficiently impeded effect of free radicals. If we disregard accidents, Aids, etc. as well as vices, such as nicotine and excessive alcohol consumption, the primary threat to our health is posed by too many free radicals, which we can stop by antioxidants.

Part IV
The Targeted Application of OPCs

Although OPCs have been proven to be a powerful substance preventing a multitude of degenerative disorders, as well as a remedy for diseases that have already manifested themselves, there are various health problems that should by no means be left to self-treatment. The ingestion of OPCs does not replace medical consultation. I strongly warn against such activities, especially if you are suffering from any kind of vascular, cardiac or circulatory disorder, oedema and diabetic retinopathy or any of the other problems listed below. Disease requires medical therapy and any self-treatment by laypersons must be supervised by a medical expert.

Protection from cardiovascular diseases

Whereas infections were the primary cause of death in previous centuries, cardiovascular diseases have attained this sad rank in the death statistics of our time. In industrialized countries, every second person dies of sudden cardiac or circulatory collapse - women as often as men.

Factors for cardiovascular diseases

- *stress*
- *smoking*
- *overweight*
- *diabetes mellitus*
- *lack of exercise*
- *excessively high levels of cholesterol*
- *hypertension (high blood pressure)*
- *chronic infections*
- *unhealthy diet*
- *predisposition*

Using OPCs to combat arteriosclerosis

Arteriosclerosis is a dreaded vascular disease caused by the gradual deposition of fat and calcium on the inner walls of the blood vessels. In the case of men, fat and calcium is deposited along the walls of the arteries leading to the heart and brain primarily between the age of 30 and 55. In women, this process starts with the menopause. These deposits prepare the ground for cardiac infarctions and strokes. Sometimes fat deposits in blood vessels can already be found in children if they consume a diet low in vitamins or live primarily on fast food products.

A healthy arterial wall is strong and elastic and adjusts to changes in internal pressure. Blood pressure varies with different levels of activity. Normally, the arteries adjust through tightening or expanding. In the presence of arteriosclerosis, however, the deposits cause them to lose their elasticity. They turn rigid and tube-like and constrict.

Let us take a closer look at the risk factors for cardiovascular diseases:

Risk factor cholesterol

In Western world most people complain - more or less panicking - about excessively high cholesterol levels. With a warning undertone, physicians announce the results of lab tests on blood lipids. The spectre of cholesterol is common talk. What does this fear-inducing term refer to? How can blood turn fatty? What is the connection between cholesterol and cardiac infarction?

For a start, cholesterol is nothing bad, but essential for life. Every day the liver produces 1000 mg of cholesterol, a fatty substance which is essential for our body cells. Once it has done its job there, it must be eliminated, but being water insoluble, it cannot travel freely in the blood stream. Water-soluble carriers called lipoproteins are needed to transport cholesterol from the liver to the cells. The elimination of used cholesterol from the body takes place in two steps: First, LDLs (low density lipoproteins) deposit cholesterol in the cells of the arterial wall. Then, HDLs (high density lipoproteins) come and pick up the deposited cholesterol and take it back to the liver. From there, it is transported out of the body via the intestines. In this way, the vessel wall acts as a temporary depot. As long as cholesterol is eliminated in this way, the amount of LDL and HDL cholesterol is balanced.

The problem begins when there are too many free radicals in the blood stream. They attack LDL cholesterol and oxidize it, preventing it from being deposited in the cells. The HDL carriers find the arterial cells empty and cannot transport the cholesterol out of the body.

Instead, white blood cells, macrophages, move into the walls of the artery and develop into foam cells, which collect the cholesterol. The more LDL cholesterol is oxidized, the more foam cells accumulate with muscle cells and calcium to form patchy deposits in the artery wall called atheromas or plaques. This makes the arteries narrower, interfering with the flow of fresh blood supplying oxygen to the surrounding tissue. When plaques rupture, the material inside gets into the bloodstream and triggers coagulation. Blood clots or pieces of plaque can block arteries, leading to heart attacks and strokes.

How can OPCs prevent atherosclerosis and an infarction? Just by being there. Strong antioxidants like OPCs help in two ways. They neutralize free radicals in the blood, which stops LDL cholesterol from being oxidized, and they keep the arteries intact by producing collagen.

Sometimes the body sends out warning signals to draw attention to imminent danger. After physical exertion you may suddenly feel excessively exhausted and feel stabbing pains in your heart and chest. In the event of such symptoms, typical of angina pectoris, you must consult a physician immediately. But such a situation should not be allowed to occur. Taking preventative measures is more prudent - and less life threatening, especially since there are so-called 'silent infarctions', which go unnoticed.

At particular risk are, besides smokers, people suffering from high blood pressure or high cholesterol levels, overweight persons, as well as all those who are genetically predisposed to cardiac disorders.

'Sparkling clean arteries':
Christa M., 52, Oehringen

Some years ago, I left hospital where I had been treated for a bad posterior myocardial infarction. The doctors informed me that the posterior cardiac artery was completely blocked, and that about 50 percent of my aorta walls were covered with deposits. While nothing could be done, it was not life threatening. I was advised to take medicine for the rest of my life. As I could not tolerate this medicine, I stopped taking it. Instead, I started taking OPCs (400 mg per day for four months, 300 mg for three months, and after that 200 mg to the present day) as well as vitamin C and some other natural food supplements.

18 months later I went back to the hospital for a check-up. A catheter angiography showed that the deposits were completely gone. 'Your arteries are sparkling clean', the stunned doctors told me. My internist could hardly believe it. 'This has never occurred before.'

OPCs and vitamin C: don't give cholesterol a chance

Tests confirm that the ingestion of OPCs provides the body with double protection against the damaging effects of cholesterol:

- Under the influence of OPCs, less cholesterol is deposited inside the inner wall of the blood vessels than when OPCs are missing from the blood.
- The cholesterol level in the blood drops, and to an even greater degree, if OPCs are taken in combination with vitamin C. Excess cholesterol is transformed into bile salts in the liver and then discharged from the body.

Especially the second item shows that no expensive drugs are required to lower the level of LDL, the 'bad' cholesterol in the blood. It is possible to tackle this problem with the help of natural substances - OPCs and vitamin C.

How to repair kilometres of cracked blood vessels?

The same applies to the fine cracks in the blood vessels, which, like calcium and fat deposits, turn into a problem with time. With increasing age, they become defective, develop small cracks and leaks and lose their elasticity. Can you imagine how laborious repair work must be in such an infinite network?

Nevertheless, there is a simple solution to this seemingly overwhelming task: If we provide the body with the two essential nutrients, OPCs and vitamin C, all the fine cracks in the vessels are repaired and everything is in perfect working order. And this applies to everybody, whether they are 25 or 70 years of age.

By doing this, we are also spared annoying and unpleasant intervention such as electrodessication. New methods, such as laser technology, are constantly being developed. But frequently, both the development and application of such techniques incur tremendous costs. All of this is unnecessary. We should focus on prophylaxis and help the body to help itself. Just dealing with the symptoms is of little use. Most diseases are caused by a lack of substances which our body is unable to produce, primarily vitamin C and OPCs. By taking these substances we enable the body to do what it can certainly achieve under these circumstances, that is to heal itself.

Headache, fatigue, lipedema, lymphedema, stress:
Nadine H., 25, Sigmaringen County

I've been taking OPCs regularly for ten months now (daily dosage of 200 mg) in combination with vitamin C. Since then, my condition has much improved.

Before, I used to have headaches several times a week. Since I have been taking OPCs, this has decreased to once a month. Although only 25 years old, I suffer from lipedema and lymphedema in my legs and have to wear elastic stockings. Now with OPCs I don't need them at work every day anymore. In the evenings my legs aren't as swollen and painful as before. My skin isn't as dry, and my hair and fingernails look better and grow faster. I have also noticed that I can work more intensively and can cope with stress better. I used to be glad to come home after work and have my peace and quiet. But now in the evenings I can still take things in and want to do things.

On the whole, I simply feel better. I can be more open and friendly because I am definitely in a better mood. I am glad to have found in OPCs something to keep me in good health.

Circulatory disorders - OPCs provide prevention and relief

OPCs for the prevention of varicose veins

Varicose veins (varices) are a venous problem. The veins take the used blood back to the heart and lungs. They are less sturdy than arteries and also have a much lower blood pressure. From the legs, the blood is pumped up to the heart where the movement of surrounding muscles pushes the blood upward. The valves of the veins prevent the blood from flowing back. Lack of exercise results in congestion. The pressure increases and under the strain the valves of the veins gradually weaken and in the end do not function at all. The blood saturated with carbon dioxide, that is waste products, stagnates in the varicose veins and does not move any further.

Varices can be clearly visible as dark unsightly swollen veins, or may remain unseen, which does not make them any less unpleasant. In the long term, they result in pain, swelling and itching. This applies particularly to haemorrhoids, which are varicose veins in the anal area. Nighttime cramps causing sleeplessness may also be the consequence of varicose veins. Usually, the only solution is surgical removal, since corrective measures are indispensable in order to prevent the development of venous inflammation, thrombosis or even varicose ulcers, i.e. open wounds along the lower legs which no longer heal.

OPCs have proven to be a helpful remedy for such conditions. In the most severe cases, OPCs are not able to completely relieve the varicose veins. But they certainly help stop new varices developing and reduce painful side effects and swelling. This effect was confirmed in various studies in 1980 and 1981.

In a test, a total of 78 persons with serious venous problems in the legs were given 150 mg of OPCs per day, a treatment that consistently brought favourable results.

Venous functional disorders of patients who did not (yet) have any varicose veins were mitigated by the administration of OPCs, i.e. OPCs proved to be a means of preventing varicose veins.

In another study, 50 patients suffering from venous problems showed considerable improvement after 150 mg of OPCs had been administered daily for a period of 30 days. The improvement induced by OPCs occurred within a shorter period and lasted longer than in a control group that was treated with other commonly used medication.

In 1985, 92 patients suffering from venous insufficiency took part in another test. After four weeks, the condition of 75 percent of the affected persons, who had ingested 300 milligrams of OPCs per day, improved noticeably. Previously described discomforts such as itching, 'heavy legs' and night-time cramps were significantly reduced.

Tumour in ankle bone:
Birgit H., 42, Scheidegg

In January 2001, I had a persistent hematoma on my upper left foot, causing me pain while walking and driving. After several orthopaedic examinations and false diagnoses, a tumour in the upper talus (ankle bone) was discovered three months later and immediately operated on.

24 hours after the operation my foot went cold. After a series of disagreeable examinations, it turned out that instead of three veins there was only one supplying the foot with blood. I should count myself lucky that my foot did not have to be amputated. Over the next 18 months I suffered from recurring paralyses, movement restrictions and strong feelings of cold in my foot.

In March 2004, I heard about a firm producing high quality micronutrients and OPCs. I grasped at this last straw and bought these products. My condition actually improved within 24 hours. I was ecstatic. Finally I could kneel beside my little daughter and play with her without worrying about not being able to get up again.

In July 2005, when hiking in the mountains, I sud-

denly felt strong pain in my left knee and couldn't walk anymore. An orthopaedist discovered that in 2001 the tumour had not been removed but only scratched. This tumour was then removed in August 2005. On the day of the operation I took micronutrients and 800 mg of OPCs, reducing this dosage daily until I reached 200 mg. Since then I have taken this same dosage every day. After ten days I could leave the hospital with good blood values and no inflammation. I have been doing sports again for one year (walking, aqua fitness, hiking in the mountains etc.). I feel perfectly fine, just like my family, who are all taking micronutrients and enough OPCs to stay healthy.

Help for haemorrhoids

Haemorrhoids are varicose veins in the anal area, which are caused by insufficient exercise. Constant sitting causes the veins in the lower intestines and the anus to expand. They start itching and may eventually burst with the risk of infection. Severe haemorrhoids, especially those inside the body, require medical treatment or surgery.

The best prophylaxis for haemorrhoids, varicose veins and veins weakened by inflammation is a healthy lifestyle involving plenty of exercise, especially swimming, walking and cycling, as well as a diet rich in roughage and essential substances. But most people find it hard to avoid sitting, due to the nature of their job. The second best prophylaxis is a sufficient supply of OPCs, which regulate the blood flow and prevent or dissolve blood clots.

Haemorrhoids:
Mr. Andreas G., 40, Munich ...

... has had similar experiences. He reported that he had been suffering from haemorrhoids for many years, had to apply stronger and stronger salves and finally ointments containing cortisone. Ever since he started taking OPCs, his condition has steadily improved. He requires almost no ointments anymore. In addition, he feels generally more vital and active.

OPCs provide relief for 'bad legs'

Although only a few scientific tests exist about the connection between OPCs and thrombosis, the idea suggests itself that the regular ingestion of an increased dosage of OPCs (200 to 300 mg/day) provides effective protection against thrombosis for persons predisposed to this ailment. It is generally known that thrombosis develops if a thrombus, i.e. a blood clot, forms in excessively viscous blood, settles at a narrow spot in the blood vessel, usually an artery, and obstructs further blood flow. Tissue that is located downstream is no longer provided with blood, which results in numerous health problems. Thrombosis assumes a particularly dangerous character

110

when the blood clot is released and migrates to the lungs, the heart or the brain where it may trigger infarction.

Since OPCs protect the inner linings of the vessels and stimulate blood flow, this substance counteracts the clotting of blood platelets and indirectly helps to guard against the dangers of thrombosis.

Swollen legs

Swollen and heavy legs are typical of vascular fragility. Lymphatic fluid extravasates from the lymph channels and accumulates in tissue, a process which results in a feeling of heaviness and fatigue as well as in swelling.

Haemorrhage

In addition to causing lymphatic fluid to collect in tissue, vascular insufficiency can also lead to haemorrhage - internal bleeding as a result of permeable veins. It manifests itself in the excessive development of bruises or the bursting of tiny veinlets in the eyes where the bleeding becomes visible as red spots.

The fact that OPCs strengthen vascular resistance has been confirmed by a number of studies:

- In 1980, a clinical study was performed involving elderly people with pronounced vascular insufficiency. The patients were suffering from burst blood vessels, senile lentigo and small, usually round, subcutaneous bleeding. Treatment with a daily dosage of 100 to 150 mg of standardized OPCs resulted in a significant improvement within two weeks. In 53 percent of the cases the result was rated 'good', in another twenty percent 'very good'.
- Another test series, where a daily dosage of 100 mg of OPCs was administered, involved 21 persons with problems of vascular resistance (Hg) and permeability. Ten of the test subjects showed significant improvement.
- In a third test series, involving patients with an average age of 46 years, vascular resistance increased from 15 cm Hg to 18 cm Hg when a daily dosage of 150 mg of OPCs was ingested.[7]

_____

7   Morton Walker: 'Medical Journalist Report of Innovative Biologics: The Nutritional Therapeutics of Masquelier's Oligomeric ProanthoCyanidins (OPCs), in: Townsend Letter for Doctors & Patients, February/March 1998, pp. 84-92

*Treating circulatory disorders in hands and feet
with OPCs*

A Dutch physician treats various disorders with
OPCs. He has had particular success in the treatment of hand and feet problems due to circulatory disorders. A tingling feeling in the extremities
and whitish-blue discoloration of fingers due to
inadequate blood flow or blue toes in elderly people, where there is insufficient blood circulation
in the extremities, are treated with alternating hot
and cold baths, ozone therapy and OPCs combined with the vitamins A and E. The doctor has
repeatedly observed that OPCs and vitamins enhance each other.

During the acute phase, he recommends 100 mg
of OPCs three times a day. Once the complaints
abate and the return of circulation to the fingers
and toes can be both seen and felt, the dosage
is reduced to 50 mg twice a day (morning and
night). Most of his patients are very comfortable
with this dosage.

Using OPCs to fight lack of concentration and learning disorders

Since OPCs pass the blood-brain barrier due to their low molecular size, they can immediately act on the brain cells and have a positive effect on lack of concentration and learning disorders. The child psychiatrist James Greenblatt from Boston, Massachusetts has systematically investigated this property of OPCs. In an interview, he declared that he used oligomeric procyanidins (OPCs) to treat concentration disorders in his clinical practice. By means of an electroencephalogram (EEG), he succeeded in identifying those aspects of concentration disorders, which could be corrected by ingestion of OPCs. He reported that this dietary supplement improved infantile lack of concentration without having any impact on the child's hyperactivity or impulsiveness. Many children suffering from concentration disorders no longer require Ritalin [conventional medication] once OPCs were administered.

James Greenblatt continued that he was initially sceptical of OPCs. But some years earlier he learned from adult patients and parents of his young patients that their concentration disorders had improved. Since they felt better, he wanted to test the preparation. In his practice, they performed EEG biofeedback analyses before and after ingestion of the drug and they examined specific brainwaves. They found that OPCs reduced the theta waves, responsible for daydreaming, and presented ten EEGs documenting the differences. James Greenblatt reported that they therefore used OPCs as a supplementary therapy for many children suffering from concentration disorders. He added that actually numerous affected adults were also easier to treat, since they did not require any medication other than OPCs.[8]

ADS: Lisbeth W., 47, France

My ten-year-old ADS son has taken 50 mg of OPCs/day for three weeks now, and he has become more attentive and altogether more positive.

Preventing the degeneration of brain cells

Brain disorders in the elderly are frequently the result of the destructive assault of free radicals, which becomes increasingly noticeable in the second half of life. OPCs pass the blood-brain barrier and have an immediate impact on the affected area in two ways: owing to their vasoprotective properties they improve blood flow to the brain as well as the condition of the capillaries, tiny blood vessels, which are responsible for providing oxygen to all cells and tissue. In addition, OPCs scavenge free radicals, which destroy the endothelial cells of small vessels.

---

8   Ibid., p. 90.

Alzheimer's disease

Memory disorders and Alzheimer's disease are the result of an insufficient supply of oxygen to the brain. If tissue is not supplied with enough oxygen, substances accumulate whose oxidation generates free radicals. If these free radicals remain unchecked, they destroy the cell walls of the nerve tissue and result in a degeneration of brain cells. OPCs are able to prevent or at least inhibit this process.

Epilepsy: Andreas S., 51, Wasserburg

I have been epileptic for 39 years. At the age of twelve I had an absence seizure for the first time. When I was 16, I suffered my first grand mal seizure, where I was unconscious for several minutes.

After that, minor and major seizures occurred again and again, imposing considerable restrictions on my life. I was unable to do A-levels and go to university as I had hoped.

My brother, four years my senior and an epileptic as well, died in 1984 after completing his studies. He supposedly stopped taking his medicine too suddenly, and the vegetal drug he took instead was totally inadequate. The exact cause of his death, however, has never been identified. Of course, I was shocked and have tried to lead a healthy life. I particularly try to eat a balanced diet.

Two years ago, I became acquainted with OPCs through

my wife. Since then, I have taken 400 mg of OPCs and, in addition, highly nutritious vitamins, minerals and protein daily. My quality of life has improved immensely since then. In conversations I am more alert and receptive. After talking with my doctor, I was able to reduce my medicine. I notice the most success, however, physically: four times a week I do Nordic Walking for one hour. Thanks to OPCs, I enjoy life more and I am very grateful.

Multiple sclerosis:
Evelyn B., 48, Bremen

Sixteen years ago, I gave birth to my daughter. It was probably then that I got multiple sclerosis. After the birth I was permanently exhausted. Yet MS wasn't diagnosed until six years ago, after I suddenly collapsed for no apparent reason. For years, I had put my chronic fatigue and exhaustion down to the exertions of everyday life. After all, I worked full-time as a secretary and, as a single mother, had to take care of my daughter and the house.

In 2001, I suffered from a series of really bad attacks. At first, the whole body was affected; then the symptoms moved to the right side. From then on, the attacks came every year and especially weakened my arm and leg. I limped and was unable to hold anything in my right hand. My eyes were affected as well. I had several inflammations of the optic nerve, which impaired my vision so much that I needed new glasses every year.

Traditional medical treatments - including interferon and vitamins in high dosages, which I did not tolerate in this form, however - relieved my symptoms, but I was too weak to work in my job anymore. After two hours at the most, I had to lie down. In the evening, I went to bed at seven or eight o'clock already. I had no quality of life anymore. In 2003, I had to retire. At that time, I was really down and became totally depressed.

Two years ago, a friend recommended OPCs, which I took, admittedly without conviction (200 mg daily with a body weight of 50 kg). After two and a half months, the doctor found amazingly good blood values during a routine examination. I gradually realized that I had more strength. Strangely enough, it was my friend who pointed out that I was staying up longer in the evenings since I had started taking OPCs. I had not noticed this connection myself. But in fact, I have made a wonderful recovery since then. Now there is scarcely any difference between my two legs. I can walk normally again, I work out regularly and I do not even have to lie down during the day anymore. Sometimes I feel like I have been re-born and it shows. At least, the people around me confirm that I look much better and seem livelier.

At the moment, I am taking part in a scientific double blind study for a newly developed MS drug. I do not know if I am actually taking this or a placebo. But I know for certain that I will continue to take OPCs along with a vegetal food supplement containing multiple nutrients and that this does me good.

Improved vision through OPCs

Retinopathy

Retinopathy is a vision impairment that affects primarily diabetics. They suffer from increased vascular permeability everywhere in the body, including the eyes. This disorder endangers not only the vascular walls but also the lens of the eye, whose gradual degeneration results in increasingly impaired vision.

The striking effects of OPCs were already tested in 1978, in a major study involving 148 retinopathy patients[9]. The administration of 100 mg of OPCs per day in addition to other types of therapy turned out to be the 'trump card' in the treatment of all vision disorders attributable to insufficient blood flow. It was irrelevant whether the impaired vision was the result of diabetes, arteriosclerosis, inflammation, degeneration, or short-sightedness.

In 1981[10] and 1982[11], similar tests were per-

---

9 Rétinopathies et O.P.C. par MM. Ph. Vérin, A. Vildy et J.F. Maurin. Bordeaux Médicale, 1978, 11, no 16, p. 1467

10 Les oligomères procyanidoliques dans le traitement de la fragilité capillaire et de la rétinopathie chez les diabétiques. A propos de 26 cas. par M. Fromantin. Méd. Int. - Vol. 16 - no 11 - Novembre 1981 - pp. 432 à 434

11 Contribution à l'étude des oligomères procyanidoliques:

formed involving 26 and 30 retinopathy patients respectively. These showed similarly positive results. In one test the test subjects were administered 100 mg of OPCs once a day; in the other test they were given 50 mg of OPCs three times a day. Their condition improved significantly. In the second study, it was possible to achieve an 80% stabilization of visual disorders.

The lens of the eye contains a lot of collagen, whose degeneration - and thus the risk of cataract development - can be prevented by regular ingestion of OPCs. As long as the opacity of the lens has not progressed too far, vision can be largely restored even without surgery.

Night blindness and fatigue due to computer monitor work

Our eyes become weaker in the course of time. We notice this deterioration when we suddenly perceive only a blurred image of objects which we used to see clearly. To a certain extent, we have to accept such age-related degenerative symptoms. But OPCs can, in principle, effect a lasting improvement to our vision, even if we strain our eyes. Continual excessive strain on our eyes results in worsening vision. This applies particularly

Endotélon, dans la rétinopathie diabétique à propos de 30 observations. J.L. Arne. Gaz. Med. de France - 89, no 30 du 8-X-1982 to people who work primarily in the dark, such as night-time cab drivers, and those who spend long hours looking at a screen, whether due to computer work, video games or television.

Macular degeneration:
Wolfgang E., Kuelsheim

My mother (69) had a macular degeneration. In January 2008 she was supposed to have an operation. Since September 2007 she has taken 100 mg OPCs daily. The day before the operation the surgeon, who was to operate the following day, came to the conclusion that the damage was not severe enough for an operation. So it was cancelled, and my mother was asked to come in April to have it looked at again.

She was again told that there was no reason for an operation, as the values had improved. The next examination was in October 2008 by the same surgeon. He couldn't believe what he now saw: The condition had improved dramatically and the macular degeneration had practically disappeared. He couldn't understand how this was possible. My mother told him that she had been taking OPCs, a purely vegetal substance. He replied that he didn't know it, but that she should go on taking it anyway. I am grateful that my mother was spared this operation at the age of 69.

Accelerated healing processes

Preventing sports injuries

Sports are a potential source of numerous injuries, some of which are related to the strength of the vascular walls in various tissue: from skin to muscles, from tendons to bones. Thus, it is necessary to strengthen these structures through regular ingestion of OPCs if you engage in sports, especially in those with a likelihood of injury. It may not be possible to prevent strain, haematomas or fractures, but under the influence of OPCs, the injury-related complaints or disorders will be less severe.

At the same time, OPCs accelerate the healing process. Wounds heal more rapidly, broken bones knit faster and haematoma recede more quickly. Collagen and elastin synthesis plays a major part in wound healing, which is the reason why this process is accelerated by OPCs. The healing process is shortened for every kind of injury: cuts and surgical incisions, burns, sprains, bruises, torn muscles and even fractures.

In 1983, a study was done involving 40 soccer players who had incurred injuries. They were divided into two groups: one half was given OPCs, the other served as a control group and did not receive OPCs. On the first day after their injury, the athletes from the first group took 400 mg of OPCs, on the next seven days they ingested 300 mg per day and on the two days after that, 200 mg per day. On the tenth day, the oedemas (injury-related swellings) were reduced more in the OPCs group than in the control group, which had not received any OPCs. In some cases the oedemas disappeared completely. The researchers also concluded that the players of the OPCs group were in better physical condition than those of the control group.[12]

More rapid healing of fractures

For prophylactic purposes the daily ingestion of 50 to 100 mg is sufficient. In the event of injury, such as fracture, the dosage can be significantly increased for a certain period, up to between 400 and 500 mg during acute disease phases.

Accelerated healing of a broken vertebra: Mrs. Gerda L., 65, from Cologne …

… fell so awkwardly from a ladder, while window cleaning, that she was unable to move and immediately knew that something terrible had happened. As a mat-

---

12 J.J. Parienti, J. Parienti-Amsellem: 'Les œdèmes post-traumatiques chez le sportif: essai contrôlé de l'Endotélon' in: Gazette Médicale de France 90, No. 3 du 21.1.1983

ter of fact, she had broken a vertebra. But she was lucky given the circumstances: no nerves had been damaged, so she would not have to spend the rest of her life in a wheelchair. At the time of her fall she had been taking OPCs regularly for one year, which she continued to do during the four torturous months of her gradual recovery. The physicians in the hospital, as well as those in the rehabilitation centre where she underwent therapy, agreed that the healing proceeded at an amazingly fast rate, which was all the more astonishing because Mrs. L.'s bones were damaged by rheumatism. Six months after her accident, Mrs. L. could move again, as though this nightmare had never happened.

Fewer oedemas following surgery

Oedemas are swellings caused by lymphatic fluid that, due to vascular injuries, extravasates into the tissue and accumulates there. They develop not only as a consequence of sports injuries, but also after certain operations, such as plastic surgery.

In 1984, 32 patients who underwent a face-lift were studied to see whether the ingestion of OPCs reduced post-operative oedemas that usually developed. From five days prior to the operation until six days after surgery, 300 mg of OPCs per day were given to half of the patients; the other 16 patients served as a control group and did not receive any OPCs. The operations were performed by the same surgeon using the same technique and under identical anaesthetic conditions.

The difference between the two groups was significant. Whereas the patients from the OPCs group had no more oedemas after twelve days, the control group took four days longer to achieve the same result.[13]

Fewer oedemas following surgery for breast cancer

After breast cancer operations oedemas often manifest themselves in the arms. This results in pain, skin tension and restricts the movement of the shoulders as well as the arms. In 1989, scientists reported that they had studied the effect of OPCs on a group of 63 women. 33 patients were given OPCs and 30 patients a placebo. During the first six weeks, the placebo was as effective as OPCs. But subsequently, the placebo effect wore off, while the condition of the group treated with OPCs continued to improve.[14]

---

13 J. Baruch: 'Effet de l'Endotélon dans les œdèmes post-chirurgicaux', in: Ann. Chir. Plast Esthét. 1984, vol. XXIX, no. 4

14 A. Pecking, J.P. Desprez-Curely, G. Megret: 'Oligomères procyanidoliques dans le traitement des lymphœdèmes post-thérapeutiques des membres supérieurs' presented at the Symposium Satellite, Congrès International d'Angiologie, Toulouse, 4-7 October, 1989

Help with joint and bone problems

In this section, I will do without any lengthy explanations and just present the testimonials of affected persons.

Arthrosis: Alexa B., 51, Sulz a/N.

I suffered from extreme arthrosis of the hips, knees and feet (hallux, great toe) for many years. The hallux of my left foot was operated on in 1980, when I was 24 years old. After that, I had to wear insoles.

At first, I felt much better after the operation, but slowly a new and very painful arthrosis developed. I could not roll my foot anymore and had a metal rolling support fitted in all my shoes. The only help orthopaedists could think of was to 'stiffen' my foot.

Finally, I found a doctor who proposed something different. He wanted to free the joint from the arthrosis by opening it up and removing the deposits. He admitted, however, that he had never done this before and, therefore, could not guarantee that it would be successful. Besides, he said it would give me only temporary, not permanent, relief.

Despite these uncertainties, I agreed to the operation. For about ten weeks afterwards I used a splint; after that I had to learn how to slowly roll my foot again. At first, it worked, but after a couple of years, as predicted, the arthrosis came back and I was in pain again.

About this time I learnt about OPCs and started taking a daily dose of 200 to 400 mg (with a body weight of 50 kg). In the beginning the result was discouraging: For about four months I felt even more pain in my feet, knees and hip. But then, all of a sudden, the pain disappeared. Now I have been trouble free for about three years and feel like a completely different person.

Pain due to missing connective vertebra: Bernd S., 44, Ludwigshafen

Since I was 13, I have suffered from massive pain in my back, the cause of which could not be determined. Injections for the pain brought no relief.

Eleven years ago, the pain was so bad that after several fruitless examinations - CAT scan, MRI and X-ray - my doctor sent me to a rehabilitation sanatorium, which, however, brought no improvement.

Four years ago, I couldn't walk standing up straight. Once again expensive examinations followed, I received injections for the pain and was sent to a sanatorium specializing in back problems in Bad Dürkheim - again to no avail.

Neither acupuncture, nor a thorough check-up at the university hospital in Mannheim helped. The doctors there thought I was just malingering. When I reacted very angrily, they offered me a special examination, which was not only very expensive but also risky. By this time, my suffering was so great that I consented to have the painful and dangerous procedure done. I might be bound to a wheelchair for the rest of my life. Fortunately, the operation went well, and this time they found something: A connecting vertebra has been missing from birth resulting in a sliding vertebra, which irritated the nerves in the spinal cord. Because of this permanent irritation the nerves get inflamed and swell. The vertebra cannot slide and squeezes the nerves, thus causing my pain. I was now offered a wheelchair, since nothing else could be done for me.

About three months ago, a colleague of mine told me about OPCs. After I had taken it daily for a fortnight (100 mg with a body weight of 75 kg), my pain stopped and I could move normally. Since then I have been without pain (!) and am infinitely happy.

Scoliosis: Carola S., Schwäbisch-Gmünd
My eleven-year-old son suffered from a scoliosis, a lateral 18 degree curvature of the spine. After he started taking vitamin C and OPCs (daily dosage of 100 mg with a body weight of 35 kg), he showed continual improvement. After six months the scoliosis improved to only 6 degrees.

Inflammation and allergies

How inflammation develops

How does inflammation develop in the body?
Damaging agents intrude into the body, attack
the organism and cause inflammation. This is the
obvious course in the event of physical injuries.
But a weakened vascular system can also be the
reason for inflammation: healthy vessels remove
intruders and prevent them from penetrating the
tissue. But if these vessels become permeable,
e.g. due to high blood pressure, they are no longer able to prevent damaging molecules from
penetrating various body tissues and causing inflammation.

Frequently, the red blood cells simultaneously
clot so that the affected regions in the body are
no longer supplied with sufficient oxygen. This
process results in an increase in destructive enzymes, which attack collagen in the cells and finally cause the cells to collapse. Destroyed vessels
result in lymphatic oedemas, i.e. a thickening of
the cutaneous and subcutaneous cell tissue, where
the lymphatic fluid stagnates. Tissue growth and
scars are another consequence of the collapse of
vascular cells.

Inflammation may also be caused directly by

free radicals. In this connection, Masquelier performed an experiment on himself in which he illustrated the strong antioxidant effect of OPCs. He applied some dithranol to two areas on his arm. This substance causes moderately severe damage to the skin by generating free radicals. In order to prove the antiradical effect of OPCs he had prepared a salve containing 0.5% OPCs. He put this preparation on one of the two areas, where he had applied the dithranol. After 48 hours, the untreated area was seriously inflamed, while the area covered with OPCs hardly reacted and had no oedemas.

How allergies are triggered

Through another reaction, this inflammation process turns into a vicious cycle. Mast cells decompose. Inflammatory substances such as histamine and bradykinin are released in major quantities. You certainly know that histamines trigger allergies. Bradykinin is a tissue hormone, which, among other things, promotes capillary permeability and thus speeds up the inflammatory process even more.

What is the function of OPCs in this complicated cycle of destruction? In 1985, Japanese scientists succeeded in furnishing evidence that OPCs were already at work where the inflammatory enzyme (hyaluronidase) is activated in the body.

In its activated state, it releases the allergy-triggering histamine, but OPCs inhibit this process. They prevent the activation of this damaging enzyme and thus play an important role in the fight against allergies.

Since these manifest themselves all over the body and in very different ways, it is clear that OPCs have a broad range of application. Before we discuss allergies in greater detail, I would like to mention some inflammatory diseases where OPCs have repeatedly resulted in amazing improvement and healing processes.

Allergies: Mrs. Hedi D., 52, Maintal

For many years I suffered from allergies to 34 different substances (among them blossoms, nuts, apples, stone fruit, perfume, washing powder, dust, bubble bath etc.) I had permanent headaches, a swollen face, itching skin and gums and also difficulty in breathing. When I was peeling potatoes, the skin of my itching and bleeding hands would crack. These problems became so bad that I could hardly eat and leave my house anymore. In the end, I had to quit my job.

After taking OPCs (200 mg per day with a body weight of 56 kg), my condition improved a lot. Only three weeks later my breathing difficulties and headaches were gone and I wasn't bothered by smells as much as before. By the end of six months I was able to eat an apple again - for the first time in ten years. When I eat stone fruit, my throat doesn't itch anymore, and the cracks in my skin are much better. My hands are fine when I peel potatoes. Now I am working in my old job again where my problems first started.'

Help with inflammatory disorders

As early as 1967, German scientists found that extracts which contain specific catechins (compounds of OPCs) are able to prevent histamine production. Since histamine is, among other things, responsible for gastric ulcers, the scientists examined the extent to which these catechin-containing extracts could be used for healing or inhibiting the development of ulcers, as well as other bleeding in the stomach. The result was self-explanatory: the administration of this extract prevented acute gastric inflammations by up to 80 percent.[15] Products of OPCs, standardized according to Masquelier's patented process, therefore have a beneficial effect on the disorders described.

Relief for all kinds of allergies

In recent years, allergies have spread in an almost epidemic manner. Some people are not even aware of their allergic hypersensitivity to

15   H. J. Reimann et al.: 'Histamine and Acute Haemorrhagic Lesions in Rat Gastric Mucosa ...' Birkhauser Verlag, Marburg University, vol. 7/1 (1977)

certain substances. These so-called allergens are frequently of animal or vegetal nature, such as plant pollen, animal fur, protein, strawberries, etc. Also chemicals, sun and water, as well as certain emotions, such as disgust or anger, may trigger allergic responses.

Free radicals play a major role in the development of allergies. The difficulty with allergies is their wide range of symptoms, which often make diagnosis and healing rather difficult. Hay-fever and asthma can be categorized as allergies relatively easily. But also arteriosclerosis, spastic bronchitis, joint and skin diseases as well as tumours may be triggered by allergens.

Allergies can have many different causes including undiscovered organic or psychic disorders. Once a psychic problem has been solved, the affected person frequently experiences significant improvement.

Since OPCs are such potent antioxidants and effectively scavenge various types of free radicals in different areas, they are recommended for allergies. Mankind has known and used their allergy-inhibiting properties for centuries without knowing what they were. The swelling and itching caused by insect bites are only the result of histamine release from mast cells. All over the world, people are familiar with common plants and grasses which can be crushed and placed on a painful spot. In France, it has long been customary to simply pick the first three leaves you find, after an involuntary encounter with the troublesome bloodsuckers. Why? Chances are relatively high that the leaves of three different plants contain enough OPCs to achieve a histamine-inhibiting effect.

There are numerous reports of affected persons who managed to cope with their allergy by means of OPCs.

Pollen allergy:
Christine H. , 58, Neckarbischofsheim

My son, 30, has suffered from a severe pollen allergy since he was three. Despite desensitization, acupuncture and every drug imaginable (I myself am a pharmacist), we never came to grips with it. Nose and eye drops as well as asthma spray were part of his life. After taking 300 mg OPCs daily for a week, he had hardly any symptoms. Later he reduced the dosage to 200 mg.

Hay fever: Petra N. , 53, Lemwerder

Since I was thirteen I have suffered from hay fever. The medicine I took in springtime always made me tired. For three years I have been taking OPCs (200 mg daily with a body weight of 57 kg) and I feel much better. I don't need medicine anymore and can even cycle through woods and meadows without getting itchy eyes, skin and throat like I used to.

Joint inflammation, neuralgia, asthma, migraines, bowel movements:
Ursula B. , 52, Sonnewalde

About 18 months ago, someone told me about OPCs. At the time I had been suffering from pain in my shoulder for nearly three years, the result of joint inflammation after a fracture. In addition, neuralgia kept me awake at night.

So I tried OPCs. In fact, after just a few weeks of only 100 mg of OPCs daily (with a body weight of 80 kg) I am so much better that I can now work in the garden again.

For 18 years I had been treated for asthma and had to take medicine regularly. A few months after I started taking OPCs, my symptoms gradually improved. This summer I only had to take my medicine if the need arose.

I have suffered from migraines for years. They are now much less frequent and weaker than before. OPCs have even had a positive effect on my bowel movements.

The targeted use of OPCs in the presence of skin problems

Neurodermatitis

This unpleasant skin disease has turned into a genuine plague and unfortunately affects an increasing number of children. It is often considered to be a multiple allergy, since it is triggered by various factors, which means it is not attributable to a clearly identifiable allergen. Another explanation is that neurodermatitis is not so much caused by allergies, but rather by psychic factors. In any case, it manifests itself in severe itching, which frequently causes afflicted persons to scratch until they bleed. This, in turn, results in infection, leading to a vicious cycle.

The therapy consists primarily of a strict diet, avoiding sweets, salt, spices, pork, fried foods (e.g. French fries), colorants and preservatives and, in some cases, milk. Such a regimen is particularly hard to explain to small children. In severe cases, cortisone is also administered, either applied topically or injected in addition, which results in severe long-term side effects.

There are no general guidelines for the treatment of this highly individual disease. Instead, each affected person has to determine the appropriate

136

regimen for him/herself. Materials that touch the skin, lots of plastics in the environment and similar factors also play an important role.

We have reports of sufferers who successfully treated this difficult disease using OPCs.

Neurodermatitis: Karla R., 10, Bielefeld

Since birth I have suffered from neurodermatitis. It comes intermittently, sometimes on journeys or in chlorinated water. Then I get itchy patches on my inner elbows or on my face. Sometimes I couldn't sleep and I scratched until it bled. My skin would itch all over my body and I had to use cortisone ointment.

Two years ago, I had acute neurodermatitis again. My parents gave me OPCs, and after two or three hours the itching and the patches were gone. When it is very bad, they give me OPCs in a high dosage (100 mg with a body weight of 25 kg).

Since then I take OPC tablets fairly regularly and I hardly ever have neurodermatitis anymore.

Eczema

Eczema is a widespread skin disease that is frequently caused by infection. It manifests itself in itching, significant reddening of the skin, as well as pimple and knot formation. When the affected areas are scratched, they turn into oozing pustules which then form scabs. Finally the scab is scratched off and the infection recurs: a vicious cycle that is hard to stop.

Since eczema is caused by contact with certain substances (e.g. solvents), it is classified as an occupational disease and can become chronic unless the affected person changes his/her profession. A strict diet or physical changes (such as puberty or menopause) may result in considerable improvement. OPCs have also been effective in the treatment of eczema.

Acne

Acne is caused by hormonal changes in the body and therefore manifests itself primarily during puberty. During this period, the skin's sebaceous glands in the face, throat and neck region produce excessive quantities of sebum. The glands become clogged and result in festering inflammation. Thus, a great number of adolescents suffer from severe pimples on their faces and throats, and that at a time when a disfigured outward appearance is perceived as particularly unpleasant.

In the case of acne, OPCs have a beneficial effect due to their inflammation-inhibiting and circulation-stimulating properties. Detoxification processes are, furthermore, accelerated. The blood flow in the skin is promoted, deep cleansing gradually results in clear and smooth skin.

Skin problems, fatigue:
Maria F., 42, Munich

Since birth my life has been overshadowed by skin problems. Bleeding hand joints, extreme itching, a terrible tight feeling in the skin all over my body, especially in my face, were everyday features of my childhood. It was neither neurodermatitis nor psoriasis. Not until years later did a doctor diagnose atopical dermatitis. Nothing helped - neither the best creams and oils, nor special diets. In the course of time my condition improved somewhat - as had been the case with my father and my aunt. The feeling was no longer unbearable, but it was not pleasant either. Somehow I managed to live with it. I had had enough of dermatologists. Stress resulted in red, sometimes also dry, patches. But these symptoms always went away again.

I have had a lot of stress since 2003. As the result of an accident I was in much pain and afraid of losing my job. My ankle joint had to be operated on a couple of times and was chronically inflamed. Two years ago, at the age of 39, I found a new job in a sanatorium which was compatible with my physical limitations at that time. Due to tension, my hands and arms had open wounds. The daily use of disinfectants didn't help, of course. In despair I used a cortisone ointment, which, however, did not help.

Fortunately, a sanatorium doctor saw my problem and recommended OPCs. Discouraged as I was at that time, I was not interested. Finally Anne Simons' book con-

vinced me to try OPCs. In January 2005, I took them for the first time - 200 mg daily with a body weight of 76 kg. I knew that I could not count on immediate positive changes. After all, the body takes time to compensate for deficits. Yet, to my surprise, one evening ten days later I discovered that my ankle joint was cool - this joint had been chronically inflamed and hot for the past three years. I could hardly believe it and watched the joint every day. Since then it has not been warm anymore, even under increased physical strain.

In addition, my exhaustion and the prevalent fatigue of the past months were reduced in the first four weeks. I have become more alert and productive, even in the evenings. In the following months, I also discovered that my marked changes of mood have decreased. I have become more balanced.

As to my skin: After exactly four months, all open wounds have disappeared. Moreover, the skin has become more tight, stable and elastic. Even though I sometimes still observe reddening in times of stress, my skin, my quality of life and my overall well-being have improved appreciably. Every day I am deeply grateful for that. I will never again do without OPCs.

Using OPCs for sunburn and damage due to radiation

OPCs apparently provide effective protection when the skin is exposed to a lot of sun or radiation. Under these conditions, free radicals multiply and attack the body with unrestrained aggressiveness. OPCs have been processed as topical preparation into a salve for topical use, which has undergone extensive testing. As a matter of fact, the ointment has also proven very effective in preventing sunburn (UV radiation). If OPCs are applied to the skin before exposure to the sun, pain and reddening can easily be prevented. Owing to their antioxidant properties, OPCs are an effective way to counter the damaging influence of the sun, a feature that has also been confirmed in medical practice.

Sunburn, radiation-related damage: Mrs. M., Netherlands

My husband personally experienced the protective effect of OPCs regarding sunburn. As he usually works indoors and spends little time outside, his skin is quite sensitive to the sun. He noticed this particularly, when he spent his vacation in a southern country. He would invariably have a terrible sunburn, despite having generously applied sun lotion. Holidays where pain prevents you from sleeping properly are, of course, anything but relaxing.

141

Being aware of the connection between the rays of the sun and free radicals, he started preparing for vacations in the sun by ingesting high dosages of OPCs. He would take between 400 and 500 mg of OPCs daily and effectively prevent the dreaded sunburns. He maintains this dosage during his entire stay.

Hormonal disorders: relieving pre-menstrual syndrome through OPCs

More and more people are complaining about a disturbed immune system as a consequence of increasing environmental stress. Many suffer from debilities and diseases which are solely attributable to the fact that their bodies fail to cope with the everyday burden of stress and pollution. A disturbed immune system also affects other body systems, such as the hormonal balance (endocrine system), which is closely linked to the emotional system.

PMS - many women suffer from this disorder

Hormonal imbalance is known to result in emotional instability and depression. Women, whose monthly cycle is subject to a complicated interplay of hormones, are particularly affected by such disorders. It is no coincidence that the abbreviation PMS has become a buzz word. PMS stands for 'premenstrual syndrome' and refers to menstrual disorders, including headache, back pain, stomach cramps as well as depression and irritability

Since OPCs boost the immune system, they are able to balance the hormonal household and so alleviate these complaints.

In a study involving 165 women suffering from PMS, the test subjects were given 200 mg of OPCs daily for four months from the 14th to the 28th day of their menstrual cycle. Within two months 60 percent of the women reported some relief from their symptoms. By the end of the fourth month, this had increased to almost 80 percent. 65 percent of the patients ceased to suffer from any menstrual pain. The ingestion of OPCs produced another pleasant result; the menstruation of women who had previously had an unpredictable cycle became more regular.[16]

This study and others came to the conclusion that OPCs alleviate menstruation, and relieve the problems which may occur during the different phases of the monthly cycle.

---

16   M. Amsellem et. al.: 'Endotélon dans le traitement des troubles veino-lymphatiques du syndrome prémenstruel - Etude multicentrique sur 165 patientes', in: Tempo Médical no. 282, nov. 1987

Headache

Many women suffer from hormone-related head-aches, which occur during, before, or after their period, but can also come between two menstru-ations. They are frequently, like migraines, per-sisting for one or two, or even more days.

Since I started taking OPCs, I have not suffered much from such headaches, although I used to experience them regularly, i.e. once a month. Other women have also told me that they have had fewer headaches since they began to take OPCs on a regular basis.

They obviously have a beneficial effect on the head in general and provide relief not only for hormone-related, but also for stress-induced headaches, as is shown by the following account.

Headaches, hot flushes:
Christine H., 58, Neckarbischofsheim

Five years ago I started taking OPCs - not because of any particular trouble, but after reading Anne Simons - I was convinced that everyone needs them. I had no idea that my regular severe headaches, which are probably due to hormonal changes, could be influenced by OPCs. For many years I had headaches during menstruation and I always needed strong painkillers. Even during menopause I suffered from headaches that occurred at times when I should have had my period. In addition, I had hot flushes that felt as if a blast furnace had been fired up within seconds. I did not want to take hormones, and other drugs scarcely helped. This was my situation when I started taking OPCs (200 mg daily). Within one week the hot flushes had gone! As soon as I reduced the dosage or had no more OPCs, the hot flushes came back again within a few days.

After about three months it struck me that I had not used painkillers for a long time. As long as I took OPCs there were no more headaches, or at least not regularly as used to be the case before. Today I can get by with 100 mg per day if necessary, but in general I take 200 mg daily (with a body weight of between 60 and 63 kg). Headaches have become the exception and I have not had a migraine since.

Enhancing the body's immune system through OPCs

Our lifestyle is marked by various strains: poisoning due to medication, excessive quantities of alcohol, heavy metals, as well as food that has been treated with chemicals which can cause trouble in the long term. Combined with increased stress factors, they all multiply the assaults of free radicals on our immune system, whose defence mechanisms are soon exhausted. Then the helpless body falls prey to a variety of disorders. We are justified in claiming that free radicals are the underlying cause of most diseases, facilitating and frequently aggravating their development, however different the disorders may be.

A 'modern' syndrome, the consequence of the immune system breaking down, is the so-called 'chronic fatigue syndrome' (CFS), which now affects millions of people, especially women over thirty or forty. Symptoms include:

- listlessness, lack of drive
- sleeping and concentration disorders
- chronic exhaustion and rapid fatigue
- depression, headache
- migrating pain in the joints
- susceptibility to infection
- swollen lymph nodes

Do you recognize some of these symptoms? It is striking that they keep recurring in reports of health recovery in individual patients after ingesting OPCs. Colds, allergic responses, concentration disorders, fatigue and lack of energy, headaches and inflamed sinuses appear in almost all cases. After the ingestion of OPCs, such symptoms normally disappear. In addition, most people report increased vitality. OPCs obviously have a stabilising effect on the immune system.

Weak immune system, cholesterol, depression: Eva L, 45., Koenigsbrunn

I've taken 100 mg of OPCs daily (with a body weight of about 55 kg) for 15 months, in addition to other vitamins. Before I started taking OPCs, my condition was characterized by chronic fatigue, exhaustion and frequent colds with a sore throat and fever, that occurred every two or three weeks. Besides, for years I had been suffering from bleeding eczema on my foot, which did not heal despite treatment with cortisone. Due to a genetically high cholesterol level (400 mg/dl), which was treated with the drug Simvastatin, I had permanently high liver values. Above all, 15 years ago I was diagnosed with reactive depression, which was treated with various antidepressants from the beginning. Since I didn't want to take drugs for the rest of my life, I made several unsuccessful attempts - after prior consultation with my doctor - to gradually reduce the antidepressants. However, as soon as I fell below a certain dosage, the depression came back so strong, that I was sometimes even unable to work. I couldn't begin to lead a normal life, not to mention feel joy.

After I started taking OPCs, my immune system clearly improved. In the first year I only had one slight cold. After about six weeks my permanent fatigue and exhaustion disappeared. With my increased vitality I experienced a quality of life which I had forgotten existed. At about this time my eczema healed completely and hasn't come back. After I had taken OPCs for about six months, laboratory findings revealed that my liver values had become normal. The cholesterol values were so good (250 mg/dl) that I could stop taking Simvastatin.

Ten months after I started taking OPCs, I tried once more to gradually reduce the antidepressants over a period of about six weeks. Thanks to OPCs I don't take any antidepressants anymore - after trying in vain to stop for 15 years. It is true that from time to time I'm subject to mood changes, but I would call these 'normal'. There is no comparison to the real depression which appeared whenever I tried to stop taking the medication before.

Tumour formation

In his U.S. patent of 1987 Masquelier mentions the influence of free radicals on tumour growth and indicates the indirect protective effect of OPCs with respect to cancer. He had already encouraged scientists to closely examine the connection between cancer and OPCs, since cancer tends to spread more rapidly in an exhausted and stressed organism. I would, however, like to fall in with Masquelier's cautious approach: 'I am aware that it is easy to raise false hopes in cancer patients.' Hence, he directs his statements about cancer to medical experts rather than to lay persons. Further research is certainly required in this respect.

Diabetes after heart operation, panic attacks: Gerhard W., Schifferstadt

In February 2005, I had a heart operation. An anterior myocardial bypass and two posterior myocardial bypasses were blocked. The long operation triggered diabetes. Three days after the operation, I had a really bad attack of tachycardia in the night. For a while I was aware of the desperate struggle of the doctors and nurses before losing consciousness.

This incident traumatized me. As soon as my heart beat became irregular, I was panic stricken, fearing another tachycardiac attack. The same happened when TV pictures of wounded people or blood reactivated the memory of this incident. I became depressive.

Three weeks after rehabilitation another attack occurred, so an emergency doctor had me admitted to hospital, where I got blood diluting medicine. I was treated by a neurologist for my panic attacks with two neuroleptic drugs. After that I calmed down.

In September 2006, I started taking OPCs (200 mg daily). After about seven weeks I reduced the neuroleptics and eventually stopped taking them. To this day I haven't needed them anymore. Since then, I have felt much better and have rediscovered a zest for life.

Part V
Beauty from the Inside: Winning the Battle against Wrinkles through OPCs

When I heard about OPCs for the first time and read initial scientific reports, I was highly interested in this 'miraculous' remedy. I was not ill, but hardly anyone can resist the promise of a slowed-down aging process. Thus, I wanted to see for myself what this supposed 'beauty from the inside' was all about. I took 150 mg a day. After three days, I found that my skin looked much smoother, or was I imagining this, because I was expecting a beautifying process? On the evening of the fourth day, I noticed to my great surprise that my terribly rough hands - I had just gone through a move and constant contact with dust and cleaning water had left its destructive traces - were suddenly perfectly smooth and soft. This effect increased during the next few days. Although I spent my days in rooms with dry, centrally heated air, my hands were so smooth and supple, that I had no need to use lotion anymore. The same was true for the skin of my entire body. Incredible. It was only then that I realized the connection with the ingested OPCs. In view of this rapid and significant response, I grew quite excited and ordered three more packages, which I gave to my mother and to two friends, strictly admonishing them to take the capsules regularly. I said no more, because I did not want to influence them. Fortunately, all three women had enough trust in me to swallow the capsules without any further explanation on my part. They soon got back to me.

They all confirmed the smoothing effect on the skin. A friend confessed that her gums had been bleeding for quite some time whenever she brushed her teeth. The bleeding stopped after she had taken OPCs for a few days.

We four 'test cases', of course, did not make up a representative group, but this was not necessary in view of the existing research literature.

One to two capsules of OPCs per day - and the skin remains young and supple

Slowing down the aging process

Can OPCs arrest or even reverse the aging process? Certainly not. But they can slow it down significantly and prevent symptoms of premature aging, both physically and mentally. This has to do with their collagen-protecting abilities.

Remember the previously employed simile of the ladder, which forms the chemical structure of collagen. The formation of rungs ensures the stability and elasticity of the connective tissue. With advancing age, crossing rungs are formed, which results in less supple, and especially in more wrinkled skin.

Just compare the tender, smooth skin of a baby with that of an elderly person. In the case of the baby, the collagen is so elastic that it protects the child from impacts. In elderly people, it has lost its elasticity, which results in degenerative symptoms and disease.

The formation of collagen requires vitamin C. OPCs enhance the effect of vitamin C and thus promote the formation of collagen. Besides they protect collagen against free radical attacks, thus significantly retarding the inevitable aging of tissues and cells.

Triple protection against aging

- OPCs regulate the 'formation of rungs' of collagen, i.e. on the one hand they ensure that the connective tissue and the vessels do not become too weak and permeable, on the other hand they prevent undesired rigidity and inflexibility.
- Vitamin C is an essential factor in the production and regeneration of collagen. If it is missing, collagen is destroyed in the body. The effects are identical to those described in the case of scurvy. As previously mentioned, OPCs are the most potent co-factor of vitamin C. Under their influence, the body requires only one tenth as much vitamin C in order to perform its tasks. Thus, OPCs ensure the development of collagen even if the body does not receive sufficient vitamin C.
- Collagen and elastin have a natural enemy in the body: enzymes. They attack the protein chains of collagen and elastin, causing the vascular walls to become brittle and excessively permeable. OPCs bond with collagen and repel this attack. The (natural) destruction of collagen by enzymes is prevented by OPCs.

You would probably like to have some evidence of the protective effect of OPCs on collagen? Masquelier also wanted such proof and performed a simple test. If immersed in hot water, collagen shrinks within ten seconds. But if the collagen fibre has been saturated with OPCs prior to immersion, it contracts more slowly and to a considerably lesser extent; to be specific, it shrinks only after 210 seconds and only one twentieth as much as the untreated collagen fibre! This test was also performed with collagen fibres that were treated with tannin, catechin and bioflavonoids respectively. OPCs did much better than any other substance. Tannin and catechin proved to be considerably less effective, and bioflavonoids obviously had no influence whatsoever on collagen stability.

OPCs literally boost the youthful appearance of our skin. They check the inevitable damage due to aging. Collagen strengthens all tissue, which is particularly visible in the skin. Furthermore, the positive effect of OPCs on elastin maintains or restores the smoothness of the skin.

Regular ingestion of OPCs ensures the youthful appearance of our skin, well beyond chronological youth. Not 'My goodness, has she grown old!' but 'She is always getting younger!' should be the normal reaction of people when they meet you after a long time.

OPCs - internal and external cosmetics

Beauty from the inside is also always beauty from the outside. The ingestion of OPCs is the most comprehensive way to improve the collagen-elastin synthesis of your skin. They can, of course, also be applied externally. The range of products containing Masquelier's OPCs also includes a topical preparation (salve in a jar). When applied externally, OPCs primarily affect the outer layers of the skin, where they ensure smoothness and elasticity, while providing protection against free radicals.

Healthy and elastic skin, basically whether your skin is dry or moist, is determined internally and depends on the nutrients supplied to the body. In this respect, the ingestion of OPCs is considerably more important than external application. Research has, nevertheless, confirmed that additional topical application of OPCs prevents inflammation and inhibits the effect of free radicals on the skin, counteracts damage due to sun exposure, and ensures smooth youthful skin.

If you consider that the cosmetics industry invests huge amounts of money in the production of salves and lotions containing collagen and promoting collagen formation, and then charges outrageous prices for such products, the cost for a package of OPCs and a jar of OPCs cream is comparably low. Ingesting just one to two such capsules daily and applying the cream on the face, neckline and sensitive areas is sufficient to ensure comprehensive collagen protection. This means that your skin is inexpensively provided with the best possible care during the day and at night, including protection against wrinkle formation, not to mention the other health benefits that OPCs have on the entire body.

.

Part VI
OPCs for Animals

The healing, regenerating and caring properties which OPCs unfold for humans are equally beneficial for animals. Particularly positive effects are achieved in wound healing and allergic processes. Since most animals produce large quantities of vitamin C themselves, OPCs are less important as its co-factor, but more significant for the regeneration of collagen.

Thus, adding OPCs to the food is an excellent method for preventing disease, slowing down the aging process, caring for the fur and accelerating the healing of wounds. OPCs have turned out to be beneficial for smaller pets and also for horses. In individual cases, excellent healing effects have been achieved.

The dosage of OPCs in animals is - similar to humans - determined by their weight. In acute cases, up to 3 mg daily are recommended per kilogram of body weight. This means that a dog weighing 20 kg would be administered up to 60 mg per day.

A cat weighing five kilograms would be given up to 15 mg of OPCs per day.

When added regularly to the food for prophylactic purposes, half the mentioned quantity is sufficient. 2 mg of OPCs per kg of body weight are considered optimal.

Open wound:
Christine H., 58, Neckarbischofsheim

For a long time my dog had an open sore on the lower edge of her nostrils, which was painful or at any rate very sensitive. Various creams were of little use as she would lick them off immediately. Our vet would have needed a tissue specimen to determine what the problem was, but I wanted to spare my dog this. Instead, for the past nine months she has been getting 50 mg OPCs daily. Her weight is between 25 and 30 kg. The open wound has nearly completely healed. While she still has an unusually dry nose, there is no open wound anymore, and she clearly feels fine.

Dog's stroke:
Petra N., 53, Lemwerder

Since OPCs worked so well with my hay fever, I decided to give them to my 16-year-old West Highland terrier when he suddenly had a stroke. It was very painful for me to watch my beloved dog suffer. He could not walk anymore and had obviously lost his sight. He seemed to have no more joy in life. I gave him 50 mg of OPCs daily (crushed and mixed with some honey) and hoped to make life easier for him. This worked. After just a short time he was able to sit up, walk and even see better. The vet encouraged me to continue with OPCs.

Appendix

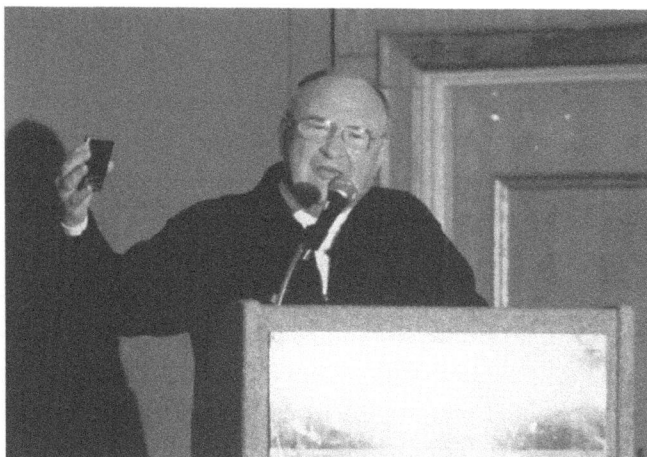

Professor's Masquelier's Speech in Baltimore on 18 October 1996

Ladies and Gentlemen,

I am very pleased to have the opportunity to speak here today, in Baltimore, before such a select audience. I hope I will be able to interest you in the story of the why, when and how, of my discovery of OPCs, the vegetable substances on which I have been working - I must admit it - for nearly half a century. But working on these substances has its charm, and does not lack a certain poetry either, because, as you see, I am beginning this lecture by showing you some beautiful flowers. *[For illustration purposes Professor Masquelier showed colour slides of plants, chemical formula etc. which he occasionally refers to in the course of his lecture.]* The substances to which I have devoted 50 years of my life, as professor and researcher, belong to the vast group of polyphenols. They are vegetable substances, and as we all know, the plant world is at the origin of the animal world, and thus, at the origin of all life on earth. In order to create life, a considerable power of synthesis is needed, so much in fact that plants are exceptionally rich in chemical components and that, when we speak of pycnogenols or polyphenols, we are immediately confronted with lists of hundreds and hundreds of components. Obviously, unless we want to end up with a veritable chemical and physiological tower of Babel, we will have to create some sort of order in these countless components.

I would, therefore, like to give you a very short course in plant chemistry, in polyphenols to be precise. Polyphenols are colored substances, or at least the polyphenols that are plant pigments are colored. Let me give you an example. This flower is red because its petals contain, what is known as anthocyanin or anthocyanic pigments, from the Greek 'anthos', which means flower, and 'kyanos', which means blue. Now you will tell me that the name is rather badly chosen, because the flower is red and the name means blue flower, but this is because the first known anthocyanin was derived from the cornflower, which is, of course, blue. One of the characteristics of anthocyans, is that they are red in acid and blue in alkaline environments. So we have to remember that the enormous group of polyphenols contains a number of red and blue pigments, the anthocyanins.

Let's now look at another group of polyphenols, the yellow pigments. Yellow, in Latin, is 'flavus', hence the name 'flavonic pigments', of which there are myriad varieties. Flavus, yellow hence flavonic pigments. Ever since these substances have been used as drugs, the word flavonic has gradually acquired a very broad meaning in pharmacy and medicine, and it has become the custom to speak of flavonoids. Flavonoid is a very handy umbrella term, but it is not quite clear what it covers. The suffix –oid denotes 'form' or 'resemblance'. Humanoid, for example, means resembling a human being. But with flavonoids, we have had the bad habit to introduce into the group large quantities of molecules that have nothing at all to do with yellow pigments. I tell you this to give you a general idea, to sort of warn you against inordinate use of the term flavonoid. One must always specify which flavonoid is meant.

In addition to the red pigments, the anthocyanins, and the yellow pigments, the flavons or flavonoids, there are a number of plants, that seem to be pigmented only by chlorophyll, the green pigment that enables leaves to perform organic synthesis. You see here before you some photographs of grape leaves. These leaves hide something truly special, namely procyanidins or proanthocyanidins, the substances on which I have been working for a great many years. They too, are polyphenols, but colorless ones. You see that the term polyphenol will fill a great big bag, a whole lumber-room full of substances and that it is absolutely necessary to be specific when talking about them. One must know whether a polyphenol is colored or not, whether it is a pigment, a blue, yellow, red pigment, et cetera, or whether it is not pigmented at all. At this very moment, Mother Nature is showing us that many green leaves turn red in autumn. The reason for this is that they contain proanthocyanidins.

There is a very simple experiment to prove the presence of proanthocyanidins. It takes an investment of, say, 30 dollars in materials, no more.

But the fact that the experiment is cheap does not make it invalid. It's also a very simple experiment to perform. You cut a grape leaf into small pieces, put these in an Erlenmeyer flask, add a diluted mineral acid, a 10-percent solution of hydrochloric acid, and heat it. While it is being heated, a red coloring will appear. After filtration, you can recover this coloring in a solution, and when you shake the solution with isoamyl alcohol, all of the red coloring will float to the top. This is how proanthocyanidins behave; or rather, how they behave in the laboratory. Whenever these proanthocyanidins are treated very intensively with a mineral acid, they transform into anthocyanins, into red pigments.

Once these proanthocyanidins have been isolated in their pure form, the experiment can be repeated in the laboratory, and each time we heat them in the presence of acid, they will be transformed into red pigment. An anthocyanin. And this is why these substances are called proanthocyanidins, because they are the precursors of anthocyanin.

It is very clear that in nature ... and I regret that being inside prevents us from seeing the beautiful spectacle nature has put on outside, although you know very well what it looks like because it is taking place under your very eyes ... a red maple forest that is taking on its typical autumn colors. But what happens in these maple leaves when they turn red in autumn? They, too, produce red anthocyanin. But this transformation has, of course, not been triggered by the addition of hydrochloric acid. And it is equally clear that, because the leaves are about to die, we do not have synthesis here but a simple transformation, the transformation of proanthocyanidins into anthocyanin. This said, we can, now phrase the problem correctly. There are two ways to demonstrate the presence of these molecules I have studied at length throughout my life. The first is in the laboratory. You take a small fragment of a plant, heat it in an acid environment and if it turns red, you have production of anthocyanin. The second is to wait patiently until autumn arrives and the leaves on the trees start turning red, and then you can say that the plant in question was secreting proanthocyanidins.

I won't bother you with the chemical formulas of these substances, I will just call to mind that these phenomena occur in plants capable of synthesizing catechins. Catechins are polyphenols, they are yet another member of the enormous and extremely complex and varied group of polyphenols. Catechins are monomers, and I will represent them here as a circle with the letter C. Some plants only synthesize catechins. A well-known example is tea. Green tea contains catechins and that's it. These catechins may vary in complexity, but they are all monomers. In other plants, however, such as the grape, the maple and a number of other plants, the catechins monomer is synthesized and then immediately bonds with itself into groups of two, three, four and sometimes five, although this is rare. These groups are known as procyanidolic oligomers or OPCs. They are the focus of my studies and I will discuss them at length today.

As you see, I have indicated catechins by the letter C. Once catechins, bonded by means of carbon-carbon bridges, have formed OPCs, they lose their identity as catechins and become procyanidolic units. For this reason, I have substituted the letter C by the letter U, so as to clearly show you that when OPCs are formed, each unit loses its identity as a catechin.

It is to show that we are dealing with something other than a condensed catechin. These catechins, bonded to each other in a U shape by means of a carbon-carbon bridge and another catechin like unit, are characterized by the fact that, when you break the carbon bridge, you do not get catechins but anthocyanins. This is the reaction I have shown you, the famous 30-dollar-experiment which may not look very serious, but which is very interesting despite its modest price, and here you see it. It demonstrates that dimers, i.e. two catechins bonded together by means of a carbon bridge, completely lose their separate identities. It is as if Miss Durand and Mr. Dupont were getting married and that, once married, no trace was left of either Dupont or Durant, but that they had taken a new name. They are still two individuals, two human beings, but the marriage that unites them has made them lose their former identity. It is important to remember that when dimers, trimers, etc. are formed, i.e. when OPCs are formed, we end up with a completely different substance. In other words, when nature decides to let a plant, tea-leaves for example, produce nothing but catechins, it will ensure that these catechins are specific. It is a mistake to talk of tannin in tea. Tea-leaves contain nothing but catechins. They may be more or less varied, but they are nevertheless all catechins. In grape leaves and maple leaves nature has decided to transform the catechins into OPCs, and has in these conditions created new individuals. Both from a chemical and from a medical or physiological point of view we must not confuse catechins with OPCs.

I will give you an example I know very well, because I come, as you know, from a region in

France where a lot of wine is produced. And very good wine too, if you'll excuse my saying so, almost as good as the Napa Valley wines. The synthesis that takes place in wine, or rather in the grape leaf, is particularly complex, because the grape leaf produces not only monomers, i.e. catechins, but also oligomers, which are, as we have seen, catechins bonded by a carbon-carbon bridge and transformed into OPCs. And then beyond these bonds of two, four, say five catechins to be generous, we get polymers. They are no longer OPCs but polymers, because beyond a certain condensation, these substances become tannins. And here, too, we must avoid possible confusion. You now see how complex the chemistry of natural substances is! The general impression is that what is natural is good, pure, simple and easily accessible. But the chemistry of natural substances is one of the most difficult kinds of chemistry to learn and remember. We should absolutely not confuse a catechin with a tannin, and that is easily done, because we speak of the tannin in tea, for example, which is a big mistake. Tea contains catechins and that's it. No tannin.

But we should also avoid thinking that there is no difference between OPCs and tannin. Tannin is an enormous molecule which, physiologically speaking, is no longer interesting. In my opinion, tannin has been used for the only valuable property it has, which has been known for a long time: its effectiveness against diarrhea. Tannins, however, are unable to cross the intestinal barrier and are therefore not bioavailable. So let's forget about tannins and concentrate on the real oligomers, small clusters of two, three, four, very rarely even five catechins bonded together by a carbon-carbon bridge and causing an anthocyanin reaction, which means that they are transformed into red pigment under the conditions I described earlier.

In 1979, I coined the word 'pycnogenol' to create a little order in this highly complex chemistry, because when we spoke of tannins, we never really knew what was what. From a chemical point of view, I coined the word 'pycnogenol' as a chemist, this word covers all these substances, because they are substances that can bond with each other under certain conditions. And the word 'pycnogenol' means in Greek: 'having the tendency to condense with itself, to create clusters of increasing complexity'. Well, you now know almost as much about this subject as I do, and if I went on about it, things would soon get very complicated and your attention would probably flag.
I will now tell you something about the research I have done, about why I am an inventor and,

in particular, why I invented OPCs for medicinal purposes. You know that an inventor does not create something out of nothing. If I were suddenly to create a white rabbit out of nothing, I would be a creator. We all know that the term creator is reserved for God, who is unbeatable in this field anyway, so it's no use trying to measure oneself with Him. The inventor is part of the universe created by God. And as we have known since Lavoisier, the great French chemist who is regarded as the father of modern chemistry, nothing in this world is created, nothing is lost, everything is transformed. So all an inventor does is transform what is already present in nature. This transformation often consists in the discovery of a new possibility of a known substance. In this sense, I was an inventor when I discovered the therapeutic qualities of OPCs, which I will turn to now.

I started my research on peanuts. Why peanuts, you will ask? Because oil is extracted from peanuts, and this was the case back in 1945. I was still a young student at the time, working on my PhD. The reason I was working on peanuts was that France had come out of the war rather badly. The United States had helped us get rid of our enemies, but the country had been bled white. We could not feed ourselves properly in France at that time. So the question was whether what remained of the peanut after its oil had been extracted, which so far had always been used to feed cattle, could not be used to feed the French? That is, provided it contained useful amino acids. So this was the problem I had been asked to tackle. In order to study the amino acids remaining in the peanut after the oil had been extracted, I had to apply an acid to reduce the proteins to amino acids. Each time I used an acid, a red color appeared. Without knowing it, I was causing cyanidolic reactions. I wanted to know what caused this red coloring, and I discovered that it was a colorless substance present in the peanut skin, a substance that originated in the peanut itself and subsequently concentrated in the skin.

In short, my doctoral thesis was gradually taking shape. This happened in 1948, on 12 July 1948, to be exact. You can work out for yourselves that I was quite young at the time, since I was born in Paris in 1922. And yet this thesis contained quite a few new facts about polyphenols. Indeed, at this time I formulated the hypothesis that these monomeric substances bond together during metabolism to form dimers by means of a carbon-carbon bridge. We had to wait fifteen years until the German chemists Freudenberg and Weinges arrived at the same conclusion and agreed with me that catechin molecules form dimers by means of this carbon-carbon bridge. This was one of the first discoveries I made at the time. The second was the following. I had been working with guinea pigs and had measured their capillary resistance after having given them this substance I had isolated from peanuts, which was, of course, an OPC, a proanthocyanidin. I noticed that this substance increased the animals' capillary resistance. But I will come back to this problem of capillary resistance later on.

The important point for me was that I did these studies at a biochemistry laboratory, obviously, but at one attached to a medical faculty. It is more or less certain that, had I been working at a laboratory attached to a science faculty, I would have limited myself to studying the chemistry of these substances. But because I happened to work at a medical faculty, I wanted to know whether these substances had any physiological importance. I was very lucky there, because I discovered that these substances had an effect on the vascular system, that they increased capillary resistance. So much so indeed that in 1950, after I had patented the method to extract these substances, the first drug based on OPCs was launched in France. It was a drug named Resivit based on proanthocyanidins derived from peanut skins. If you came to France on a visit and walked into a drugstore, you could ask for Resivit and they would be glad to sell it to you. Of course they would, that is how they make their money, but it shows that this vascular protector Resivit has been on sale in France since 1950 and is still on the market. The peanuts used to make Resivit were imported from Africa in their shells. Shortly after the introduction of Resivit, however, the peanuts started arriving in Bordeaux without their shells. The Senegalese had started shelling them using this simple gadget and henceforth, they arrived in Bordeaux without their skins. This meant that our source of raw material for the drug had dried up and I had to find another source of OPCs. I happened to find it in the pine forest near Bordeaux, which stretches from the south of the city all the way to the Spanish border. The region is called 'Les Landes', and in the bark of the pine trees from this region I found proanthocyanidins, OPCs, once more. I undertook the study of it and discovered a method to extract it. This extraction method was the object of the patent I registered in 1951. As you see, all this goes back quite a long way and it clearly establishes that people in France were interested in this substance at the time, or at least that some people in Bordeaux and at my laboratory were.

This patent was at the basis of Flavan, a drug based on pine bark OPCs. They also have an effect on the vascular system. Hence, Flavan is also a vascular protector. It is still on sale in French drugstores and is still being prescribed by French doctors.

To continue with the positive results of my research, about ten years later we, at my laboratory, came up with the idea of analyzing grape seeds. We discovered that the OPCs present in the grape leaf migrated from the leaf to the grape seed and concentrated there. This made grape seed a very interesting raw material for the extraction of OPCs, especially because it was cheap and plentiful, being a by-product of Bordeaux wine production. During the grape harvest, when the grapes are in and have been pressed, you will find veritable mountains of grape seeds. Grape seeds are sometimes used for oil extraction, because grape seed oil is excellent, a delicious edible oil, rich in polyunsaturated fatty acids. But they cannot all be used for oil extraction, there are far too many, so the industry began to use them also as a new source of OPCs. In a grape seed, the oil is on the inside; on the outside is a zone containing tannin and right on the surface of this tannic zone are the OPCs.

The tangible result of all this is the third drug, Endotélon, another vascular protector, based on grape seeds left over from the Bordeaux wine-making process.

As you see, it has been a continuous process through the decades, a process of development of three drugs based on natural substances all with the same therapeutic profile, i.e. protection of the vascular system. But how does one establish this protective effect on the vascular system? By measuring the resistance of the small capillary vessels. Capillary resistance is simple to measure. All you have to do is make a vacuum in this glass vial with this little piece of equipment, and you can measure the depression that has been created with a manometer, in centimeters of mercury. To perform the measurement, you apply the equipment to the skin and draw a vacuum until tiny little hemorrhages appear. The measurement that you see here has been performed at a depression lower than capillary resistance, but if you create a depression equivalent to 25 centimeters of mercury on the manometer, which is generally the required depression for a healthy human male, the first capillaries will start to burst, and you will have measured capillary resistance. This measurement can, of course, also be performed on guinea pigs or other animals.

What happens under the skin during this measurement? Quite simply, the capillaries burst. Here you see a picture of a burst capillary taken with an electron microscope. You see the red blood cells, the lymphocytes, the interior of the capillary, the cells surrounding it and something else that is worth noticing because it acts more or less like wrapping tissue around the cell wall: collagen fibers.

And with this, I have reached the most essential element of my new discoveries on OPCs at the time, their effect on collagen. One might say that since my publication of this encompassing table, proanthocyanidins, OPCs, can be considered as 'collagen vitamins', because they partake in the biosynthesis of collagen and prevent its destruction. Let's first of all look at biosynthesis. As you know, the biosynthesis of collagen requires ascorbic acid, vitamin C, because the amino acids proline and lysine must be hydroxylated before they can be incorporated as physiologically active collagen. The OPCs act as cofactor of vitamin C, reinforce its effect and thus activate collagen production. You can compare this to repairing a broken ladder with only two rungs left. It must be repaired and given new rungs. Thanks to the OPCs, the collagen reinforces itself by means of cross-links, which renders it once again functional, physiological, and solid, as in the image of the repaired ladder.

But I need not tell you, ladies and gentlemen, that you cannot repair a ladder with no matter what kind of piece of wood. The pieces of wood must have the right size and must fit between the two uprights. If you use pieces of wood that are too long, your ladder will turn out all crooked and be useless. I use this image to make it clear that if you were to use a tannin or, on the other hand, a catechin, you would be using pieces of wood that were too big or too small and would never fit between the uprights. The uprights of the ladder are the collagen fibers, and here you have, for example, a polyphenol that wants to insert itself between the uprights of the ladder. These polyphenolic substances must have a certain molecular size if they are to repair the collagen. OPCs happen to have the right size to fit perfectly between the collagen fibrils. You can measure this by the contraction of a collagen fiber immersed in hot water. As soon as the hot water is turned on, the collagen fiber contracts. We see this very well by means of the rapid contraction of the reference fibers. The same is true of fibers that have first been brought into contact with what I would call 'ordinary' bioflavonoids. With catechins, the contraction is somewhat delayed, which means that the collagen is a little stronger. And even though tannins provide an even longer delay, the longest contraction time is obtained with OPCs. The longer the contraction time, the better the collagen has been repaired. Here you see once more a confirmation of the fact that you need molecules of a particular size for the repair to be carried out. You cannot use just anything to repair decayed collagen.

My laboratory performed other experiments with guinea pigs, to prove that OPCs are cofactors of vitamin C. We experimented with four batches of guinea pigs. The first batch was deprived of vitamin C entirely. They survived for about 5 weeks and then died of scurvy. A control batch was given a well-balanced diet with plenty of vitamin C and they not only survived but gained weight in the course of the experiment. But we discovered something very interesting in the other two batches of guinea pigs, which were given a little vitamin C, but not enough to survive. This is the curve you get when you feed the animals a little vitamin C, but not enough to keep them alive. They die after about 9 weeks. However, if you give guinea pigs the same insufficient quantity of vitamin C but this time with added OPCs, they survive. By adding OPCs to the ascorbic acid, its effect is prolonged and reinforced. You might therefore say that OPCs are cofactors of ascorbic acid. And there is no better way of demonstrating the beneficial effect of OPCs on vitamin C. Here … I will go over this very quickly … you see evidence that OPCs inhibit enzymes that destroy collagen, such as elastase, and in general inhibit enzymes that attack proteins. Finally, returning to the preceding table, we see that it is under these conditions that proanthocyanidins play a role in the construction of collagen and inhibit its destruction by enzymes that accelerate collagen destruction, such as collagenases. As you know, there are certain diseases, known as collagen diseases, that are characterized by hyperactivity of these destructive enzymes. These experiments proved the therapeutic effect of OPCs on the circulation. Given that the wall of a blood vessel, the endothelium, is full of collagen, which ensures the elasticity and resistance of the vessel, it follows that by protecting the collagen, by improving the quality of the collagen, you also improve the quality of the vessel itself.

We also had to prove the OPCs were bioavailable. And this was not at all self-evident, because polymerized OPCs begin to resemble tannins, and we knew that tannins were not bioavailable. Tannins taken orally do not cross the intestinal barrier. How would we prove that OPCs do cross this barrier? In other words, how to prove that OPCs taken orally, whether by an animal or a human being, would end up more or less everywhere inside the body? To achieve this, we marked grape OPCs with radioactive carbon 14. Of course, we could not mark the pine trees of the Les Landes region, since we could not take them to our laboratory, so we grew 'mini-vines' instead. These we kept in an atmosphere of carbonic acid for 45 days, using radioactive carbon 14. Photosynthesis continued for 45 days and in particular the OPCs synthesized with the radioactive carbon. After 45 days, when we picked the leaves from the vines and placed them on photographic paper in the dark, we obtained 'auto X-rays': the grape leaves were radioactive and photographed themselves. So, if you feed an animal proanthocyanidins, OPCs derived from grape seeds treated with radioactive carbon, their distribution inside the body becomes measurable by the radioactivity emitted by each of the animal's organs, as you see on this table. In this table, we have set the blood total at 1, and you see that the aorta is most radioactive at the same time. If the blood's total radioactivity is set at 1, that of the aorta is 7 or 8 times higher. This first of all means that OPCs spread throughout the body but have a particular affinity for the vascular system.

If you take a slice of the animal, this is a cross-section of a mouse frozen in liquid helium, and place it on radiographic film, all the patches that show up white are radioactive. Here is the cross-section of the aorta, for example, and the skin. In short, radioactivity is spread throughout the body, which proves that OPCs are bioavailable. Here you have the radioactivity on a blowup of the animal's heart, and you see how much the OPCs do indeed attach themselves to the collagen in the walls of the arteries that transport the blood to and from the animal's heart.

It is far from self-evident that other polyphenols are also bioavailable. I have already indicated that tannins are not, and there is another polyphenol named rutin or rutoside that is widely sold as a food supplement. And I am sure it has some activity, I don't doubt it, but when we marked rutoside with carbon 14 as we had done for the grape seed OPC and fed it to an animal, the only radioactivity we could detect was in the digestive tract. Obviously, the rutoside had to be somewhere, but it had remained inside the intestine. We had to pencil in the outline of the animal's body, because only the intestine was radioactive, nothing else. This proves that this flavonoid is not bioavailable. It is still on sale as a medicine, which is of course very nice for those who sell it, but it has not been proven like OPCs.

I am now coming to the final part of my lecture, which I will shorten so as not to abuse your patience. As you will remember, my first work was on peanuts. Peanuts contain oil and, as if by chance, this oil is enveloped in a skin that contains OPCs. I subsequently worked on the pine tree from the Les Landes region, which contains a resin that is very sensitive to oxidation, and, as if by chance, this resin is also protected by a sort of 'bark shell' very rich in OPCs. Thirdly, I turned to grape seeds. I have already told you that grape seeds contain an oil that is very rich in polyethylenic fatty acids, and lo and behold, grape seeds, too, are surrounded by a zone rich in OPCs. In brief, plants take the precaution to surround themselves with OPCs if they have to protect themselves from oxidation. Why should we humans not do the same? We, too, have reason to fear the effects of oxygen. I asked myself this question, and in trying to answer it I discovered the particularly powerful protective effect of OPCs against the free radicals of oxygen.

This is a photo of a book. This book from my library is a hundred years old and like all old books, it has turned yellow. Despite careful handling, oxygen has caused the paper to turn yellow, as everyone can see for themselves. Something else everyone can easily check themselves is the following.

Take a page from a newspaper and put it outside in the mid-day sun on a fine summer's day, after first having placed an opaque plate in the center of the paper. Leave the paper exposed to the sun for three hours. After three hours, you will find that the paper has yellowed almost as much as the book has in a whole century. So what happened? The paper has clearly not turned yellow underneath the plate where it was protected from the sun. It means that oxygen reinforced by sunlight tends to transform into free radicals. In other words, molecular oxygen becomes the radical superoxide and woe to the molecules that stand in its way, because they stand a fair chance of being broken into pieces. The effect of all this on collagen is clear from this picture of an old peasant woman from the mountains of Peru. You don't need me to tell you that this is an example of seriously deteriorated collagen in someone who has passed more than sixty years at high altitudes and has therefore been exposed not only to oxygen, but also to sunlight and free radicals.

All this is rather commonplace and very well known. But we might be led to believe that it only concerns the outside of our bodies. Well, it doesn't. Each cell in our body has to eliminate molecules, and cells generally use oxygen to eliminate molecules they have no use for, awkward molecules they do not want inside their cytoplasm. However, some of these molecules cannot be eliminated by the molecular oxygen we breathe. Our own bodies transform part of the oxygen into free radicals. Indeed, we have inside our bodies free radicals we produce ourselves in order to rid the interior of our cells from substances such as 'capital X' that cannot be oxidated by the normal oxygen we breathe. So you see that free radicals have a physiological role. Incidentally, 'X' could be alcohol. Alcohol is one of the substances that require free radicals to be removed from our cells. All this is hardly consoling, but we do have certain natural defenses. The way our body uses free radicals to detoxify its cells is a bit like killing a fly with a Kalashnikov. Effective, certainly, but the damage to everything around the fly is substantial. So, to prevent this 'overkill' we have protective systems in the form of enzymes, such as super oxide dismutase, Glutathion peroxidase, catalase. They prevent the initial reaction by the super oxide molecule from turning into a chain reaction; they prevent the production of the super oxide from being followed by a whole host of free radicals. All this works very well, but … these enzymes are proteins, and with age our capacity to synthesize proteins decreases. Besides age, there are genetic defects that affect our capacity to synthesize proteins.

Now you will say: 'But surely there are vitamins,

vitamin E, vitamin C. They are antioxidants that play a role in our natural defense system.' They do indeed, but only if we eat food that contains enough of them! And we cannot always check the doses of vitamin C and E we consume in a day. And then there is the extremely unhealthy modern practice of strict dieting that often causes a highly insufficient vitamin consumption. The result is that many people produce an excess of free radicals. We can thank our lucky stars for the existence of radical scavengers, substances that help us fight free radicals. These substances are OPCs. I will prove it to you. This is DPPH, diphenyl-picryl-hydrazyl, a free radical. If, little by little, you add OPCs, proanthocyanidins, for example, to the DPPH, radical activity will disappear. Here you see the DPPH without OPCs, with a little OPC and with sufficient OPCs to ensure complete suppression of radical activity. All this can be observed with the naked eye. Here you have the free radical, which is colored, and which slowly loses its color and disappears as we add more OPCs to the solution.

You may object that this is all very well, but that it only happens 'in vitro', that it is not real. So the question is, does this really happen in our bodies? I have already demonstrated that OPCs are bioavailable and are absorbed into our tissues. So I carried out an experiment, using my-self as a guinea pig. I applied some dithranol, a substance that produces free radicals, on my arm. Forty-eight hours later, the skin of my arm showed the lesions characteristic of the action of free radicals, unless I applied a small quantitiy of a cream based on OPCs derived from grape seeds five minutes after applying the dithranol. You see here that the reaction to the radicals is much weaker. This proves that the antiradical ac-tion also occurs in living tissue.

All this has led to my registering this patent in 1987. A US patent that was granted to me for a 'plant extract with a proanthocyanidins content, as therapeutic agent having radical scavenger ef-fect, and use thereof.' I must say that this pat-ent has not been received with unbounded joy in some circles in this country. Some people won-dered where I got the cheek to register a patent under their very noses, as it were. But that's how it was. If you have been doing research for 40 years, I'd say you have a right to register a few patents. And I have registered patents all over the world. Anyway, the US patent office in Washing-ton has been so kind as to grant me this patent, and I am very proud to be holder of a United States patent for this discovery. This is to show you that the cosmetics industry, both here and in

France, makes use of anti-radical substances. In France we have a whole line of cosmetics containing pycnogenols derived from grape seeds.

A few final words on the 'French Paradox'. I promise I will be brief. You see here the photo of a paper I published in 1961. In it, I argued that wine lowered cholesterol thanks to the 'flavonic derivatives' it contains. This is how we called proanthocyanidins at the time. The word proanthocyanidins was not coined until 1970, so in 1961 we still called them flavonic derivatives. I presented this paper at an international medical conference on the use of wine and grapes. Among my audience was the Dean of the Faculty of Medicine of UCLA, Milton Silverman. When I had finished, Mr. Silvermann stood up and said: 'Dear Professor, please come and give this lecture at UCLA, I am sure it will be a great success. Because at the moment,' - we are talking 1961, - 'there are two things Americans fear most of all: communism and cholesterol.' I end this talk by showing you that the 'French Paradox' was already an integral part of my work in 1961.

Thank you for your attention.

Literature

Agarwal C. et al.: 'A Polyphenolic Fraction from Grape Seeds Causes Irreversible Growth Inhibition of Breast Carcinoma MDA-MB468 Cells by Inhibiting Mitogen-activated Protein Kinases Activation and Inducing G1 Arrest and Differentiation', in: Clinical Cancer Research, 2000, 6 (7), pp. 2921-30

Alberto, M.R.: 'Antimicrobial effect of polyphenols from apple skins on human bacterial pathogens', in: Electron. J. Biotechnol., 2006, 9 (3) Valparaíso, online-version

Amsellem, M. et al.: 'Endotélon dans le traitement des troubles veino-lymphatiques du syndrome prémenstruel - Etude multicentrique sur 165 patientes', in: Tempo Médical no. 282, nov. 1987

Baruch, J.: 'Effet de l'Endotélon dans les œdèmes post-chirurgicaux. Résultats d'une étude en double aveugle contre placebo sur trente-deux patientes', in: Ann. Chir. Plast. Esthét. 1984, vol. XXIX, no. 4

Belcaro G. et al.: 'Treatment of osteoarthritis with Pycnogenol. The SVOS (San Valentino Osteo-arthrosis Study). Evaluation of signs, symptoms, physical performance and vascular aspects', in: Phytother Res., 2008, 22(4), pp. 518-523

Belcaro G. et al.: 'Pycnogenol® improvements in asthma management', in: Panminerva Medica 53 2011, 3 Suppl. 1, pp. 57-64

Belcaro, G. et al.: 'Improvement in signs and symptoms in psoriasis patients with Pycnogenol® supplementation', in: Panminerva Medica 56 (1) 2014, pp. 41-48

Belcaro, G. et al.: 'Pycnogenol® improves cognitive function, attention, mental performance and specific professional skills in healthy professionals aged 35-55', in: Journal of Neurosurgical Sciences, 2014, 58(4), pp. 239-48

Belcaro, G. et al.: 'The COFU3 Study. Improvement in cognitive function, attention, mental performance with Pycnogenol® in healthy subjects (55-70) with high oxidative stress', in: Journal of Neurosurgical Sciences, 2015, 59(4), pp. 437-46

Beylot, C., Bioulac, P.: 'Essai thérapeutique d'un angioprotecteur périférique, l'Endotélon', in: Gaz. Méd. de France 87, No. 22 du 13/6/1980

Cao, A.H. et al.: 'Beneficial clinical effects of

grape seed proanthocyanidin extract on the progression of carotid atherosclerotic plaques', in: Journal of Geriatric Cardiology (JGC), 2015, 12(4), pp. 417-423

Cesarone, M.R. et al.: 'Kidney flow and function in hypertension: protective effects of pycnogenol in hypertensive participants - a controlled study', in: Journal of Cardiovascular Pharmacology and Therapeutics, 2010, 15(1), pp. 41-46

Chayasirisobhon S.: 'Use of a Pine Bark Extract and Antioxidant Vitamin Combination Product as Therapy for Migraine in Patients Refractory to Pharmacologic Medication', in: Headache 2006, 46(5), pp. 788-793

Diedrich, C.M., Simons, Anne: Das Teebaumöl Praxisbuch. Bern, Munich, Vienna 1996

Frankel, E.N. et al.: 'Inhibition of oxidation of human low density lipoprotein by phenolic substances', in: The Lancet, 1993, 341, pp. 454-457

Grossi, M.G. et al.: 'Improvement in Cochlear Flow with Pycnogenol® in patients with tinnitus: a pilot evaluation', in: Panminerva Med. 2010, 52 (2 Suppl 1), pp. 63-67

Hertog, M.G.L. et al.: 'Dietary Antioxidant Flavonoids and Risk of Coronary Heart Disease', in: The Lancet, 23. Okt. 1993

Hosseini, S. et al.: 'A randomized, double-blind, placebo-controlled, prospective, 16 week crossover study to determine the role of Pycnogenol in modifying blood pressure in mildly hypertensive patients', in: Nutrition Research, 2001, 21(9) pp. 1251-1260

Hughes-Formella, B. et al.: 'Anti-inflammatory and skin-hydrating properties of a dietary supplement and topical formulations containing oligomeric proanthocyanidins', in: Skin Pharmacol Physiol., 2007, 20(1), pp. 43-49

Jones, Frank: Mit Rotwein gegen Herzinfarkt. Cologne 1996

Kenny, Thomas P. et al., 'Immune Effects of Cocoa Procyanidin Oligomers on Peripheral Blood Mononuclear Cells', in: European Journal of Pharmacology, 2013, 714(1-3), pp. 218-228

Kilham, Chris: OPC The Miracle Antioxidant. How it acts to prevent disease, restore health and upgrade quality of life. New Canaan, Connecticut 1997

Kohama, T., Negami, M., 'Effect of low-dose French maritime pine bark extract on climacteric syndrome in 170 perimenopausal women: a randomized, double-blind, placebo-controlled trial', in: J Reprod Med. 2013, 58 (1-2), pp. 39-46

Laparra, J., Masquelier, J., Michaud, J. : Action des Oligomères Procyanidoliques sur le Cobaye Carencé en Vitamine C. Travaux originaux. Université de Bordeaux 1976

Leger, A.S.St. et al.: 'Factors Associated with Cardiac Mortality in Developed Countries with Particular Reference to the Consumption of Wine.' The Lancet, 12 May 1979

Liu X. et al.: 'Pycnogenol®, French maritime pine bark extract, improves endothelial function of hypertensive patients', in: Life Sciences 74, 2004, pp. 855-862

Luzzi R. et al. 'Pycnogenol® supplementation improves cognitive function, attention and mental performance in students', in: Panminerva Med., 2011, 53 (3), pp. 75-82

Luzzi R. et al: 'Normalization of cardiovascular risk factors in peri-menopausal women with Pycnogenol®', in: Minerva Ginecol. 2017, 69 (1), pp. 29-34

Luzzi, R. et al.: 'Improvement in symptoms and cochlear flow with Pycnogenol in patients with Meniere's disease and tinnitus', in: Minerva Med, 2014, 105 (3), pp. 245-54

Marini, A. et al.: 'Pycnogenol® effects on skin elasticity and hydration coincide with increased gene expressions of collagen type I and hyaluronic acid synthase in women', in: Skin Pharmacology and Physiology 2012, 25 (2), pp. 86-92

Masquelier, Jack: 'Action protectrice du vin sur l'ulcère gastrique', in: Résultats, p. 61

Masquelier, Jack: 'Premier American Scientific Address', Speech in Baltimore on Oktober 18, 1996

Masquelier, Jack, Schwitters, Bert: A Lifetime Devoted to OPC and Pycnogenols. Jack Masquelier's pioneering and innovative role in the isolation, identification and application of oligomeric proanthocyanidins / OPC. Rome 1997

Ni, Z., Mu, Y., & Gulati, O.: 'Treatment of melasma with pycnogenol', in: Phytother Res (16), 2002, pp. 567-571

Parienti, J.J., Parienti-Amsellem, J.: 'Les œdèmes post-traumatiques chez le sportif: essai contrôlé de l'Endotélon', in: Gazette Médicale de France 90, No. 3 du 21.1.1983

Pecking, A., Desprez-Curely, J.P., Megret, G.: 'Oligomères procyanidoliques dans le traitement des lymphœdèmes post-thérapeutiques des membres supérieurs', presented at the symposium Satellite,

Congrès International d'Angiologie, Toulouse, 4.-7. Oktober 1989

Reimann, H. J. et al.: 'Histamine and Acute Haemorrhagic Lesions in Rat Gastric Mucosa: Prevention of Stress Ulcer Formation bei (+)-catechin, an Inhibitor of Specific Histidine Decarboxylase in vitro', in: Agents and Actions Bd. 7/1, Birkhauser Verlag., University of Marburg, Vol. 7/1 (1977)

Sano, Atsushi et al.: 'Proanthocyanidin-rich grape seed extract reduces leg swelling in healthy women during prolonged sitting', in: Journal of the Science of Food and Agriculture, 2013, 93 (3), pp. 457-462

Sarrat, L.: 'Abord thérapeutique des troubles fonctionnels des membres inférieurs par un microangioprotecteur l'Endotélon', in: Bordeaux Méd. 11, 1981, pp. 685-8

Schwitters, Bert (with Prof. Jack Masquelier): OPC in Practice. The Hidden Story of Proanthocyanidins, Nature's Most Powerful and Patented Antioxidant. Rome 1995 (2nd Vol.)

Schwitters, Bert: 'Masquelier's TM Original OPCs and 10 grape seed extracts. An Independent, Reproducible State-of-the-art Comparative Analysis': Special Inc. Report, U.S.A. November 1997

Schwitters, Bert: Dr. Masquelier's Mark on Health. Rome 2004

Simons, Anne: Das OPC-Arbeitsbuch. Coburg 2004

Simons, Anne: Frauen leben länger mit OPC. Munich 2018

Simons, Anne: Cholesterin senken mit OPC. Munich 2021

Simons, Anne: Das Schwarzkümmel Praxisbuch. Bern, Munich, Vienna 1997

Simons, Anne: Öle für Körper und Seele. Wundermittel der Natur. Das umfassende Praxisbuch. Munich 1997

Simons, Anne: The Bible of Natural Healing Agents. Munich 2001

Simons, Anne: Maya-Medizin. Munich 2000

Simons, Anne: Die Kunst der Selbstverjüngung. Ganzheitliches Anti-Aging. Munich 2004

Sung, N.Y. et al: 'The procyanidin trimer C1 induces macrophage activation via NF-ϰB and MAPK pathways, leading to Th1 polarization in murine splenocytes', in: Eur J Pharmacol. 2013, 714, pp. 218-28

Suzuki, N. et al.: 'French maritime pine bark extract significantly lowers the requirement for analgesic medication in dysmenorrhea: a multi-center, randomized, double-blind, placebo-controlled study', in: J Reprod Med. 2008 May, 53 (5), pp. 338-46

Takahashi, T. et al.: 'Proanthocyanidins from grape seeds promote proliferation of mouse hair follicle cells in vitro and convert hair cycle in vivo', in: Acta Derm Venereol 1998 Nov, 78 (6), pp. 428-32

Trebatická J. et al.: 'Treatment of ADHD with French maritime pine bark extract, Pycnogenol', in: Eur Child Adolesc Psychiatry, 2006, 15 (6), pp. 329-35

Uchida, Edamatsu et al.: 'Condensed tannins scavenge active oxygen free radicals', in: Med. Sci. Res. (15) 1987, pp. 831f.

Vinciguerra G. et al.: 'Cramps and muscular pain: prevention with Pycnogenol® in normal subjects, venous patients, athletes, claudicants and in diabetic microangiopathy', in: Angiology, 2006, 57, pp. 331-339

Vogels, Neeltje et al.: 'The effect of grape-seed extract on 24 h energy intake in humans', in: European Journal of Clinical Nutrition, 2004, 58, pp. 667-673

Walker, Morton: 'Medical Journalist Report of Innovative Biologics: The Nutritional Therapeutics of Masquelier's Oligomeric Proanthocyanidins (OPCs)', in: Townsend Letter for Doctors & Patients, Feb/Mar 1998, pp. 84-92

Weseler, Antje R. et al.: 'Pleiotropic benefit of monomeric and oligomeric flavanols on vascular health - a randomized controlled clinical pilot study, PLoS ONE 2011, 6 (12)

Wilson, D. et al.: 'A randomized, double-blind, placebo-controlled exploratory study to evaluate the potential of pycnogenol for improving allergic rhinitis symptoms', in: Phytother Res., 2010, 24 (8), pp. 1115-9

Worm, Nicolai: Täglich Wein. Gesünder leben mit Wein und mediterraner Ernährung. Bern and Stuttgart 1997 (4th vol.)

Yamakoshi J. et al.: 'Oral intake of proanthocyanidin-rich extract from grape seeds improves chloasma', in: Phytother Res., 2004, 18 (11), pp. 895-99

Yang, H-M. et al., 'A randomized, double-blind, placebo-controlled trial on the effect of Pycnogenol® on the climacteric syndrome in peri-menopausal women', Acta Obstet Gynecol Scand, 2007, 86, pp. 978-985

Zandi, P. et al: 'Reduced risk of Alzheimer disease in users of antioxidant vitamin supplements: the Cache County Study', in: Arch Neurol, 2004, 61(1), pp. 82-88

Notice

Professor Dr. Jack Masquelier, discoverer and leading authority in the field of OPCs research, has developed the basis for a standardized process that ensures that the OPCs content is highly concentrated and always of consistent, first-class quality. Such products are constantly tested for purity and quality; only they are authorized by him. According to the information available to me, there is no risk involved in buying products containing OPCs from the International Nutrition Company (INC) (www.masqueliers.com).

www.ingramcontent.com/pod-product-compliance
Ingram Content Group UK Ltd.
Pitfield, Milton Keynes, MK11 3LW, UK
UKHW041629010825
7193UKWH00009B/58